CNA Exam Practice

Review Questions for

The Nurse Assistant Exam

Key Points Exam Prep Team

CNA Exam Practice

Review Questions for The Nurse Assistant Exam

ISBN-13: 978-1545082997

ISBN-10: 1545082995

Printed in the United States of America.

Section 1

Hospitals and nursing centers

1. .... is a nurse who has completed a 1 year nursing program and has passed a licensing test
   a. Registered nurse
   b. Licensed practical nurse
   c. Nursing assistant
   d. Director of nursing

2. .... is an illness or injury from which the person will not likely recover
   a. Chronic illness
   b. Acute illness
   c. Terminal illness
   d. Severe illness

3. Which of the following is a health care agency or program for persons who are dying?
   a. Assisted living residence
   b. Hospice
   c. Old people's home
   d. Care home

4. A nurse who has completed 2 to 4 years nursing program and has passed a licensing test is known as
   a. Registered nurse
   b. Licensed vocational nurse
   c. Licensed practical nurse
   d. Nursing assistant

5. Which of the following is a characteristic of chronic illness?
   a. It can be controlled
   b. It has no known cure
   c. It is slow or gradual in onset
   d. All of the above

6. Which of the following is an example of acute illness?
   a. Heart attack
   b. Diabetes
   c. Cancer
   d. All of the above

7. All of the following services can be provided in a long term care center EXCEPT
   a. Social services
   b. Recreational services
   c. X ray procedures
   d. Medical services

8. A disability occurring before the age of .... is called developmental disability.
   a. 2 years
   b. 10 years
   c. 20 years

d. 22 years

9. Which of the following persons can be admitted to a long-term care center?
   a. Terminally ill persons
   b. Mentally ill persons
   c. Alert and oriented persons
   d. All of the above

10. ……………provides housing, personal care, support services, health care, and social activities in a home like setting for persons needing help with daily activities
    a. Hospice
    b. Assisted living residence
    c. Hospitals
    d. All of the above

11. ….. is complex medical care or rehabilitation when hospital care is no longer needed
    a. Subacute care
    b. Extended care
    c. Dementia care
    d. All of the above

12. Patients in hospices usually have about ……….. to live
    a. 6 months
    b. 2 years
    c. 5 years
    d. 10 years

13. A hospital has a governing body called ………..
    a. Management team
    b. Heads of departments
    c. Board of directors
    d. Health team

14. Which of the following is a function of the board of trustees
    a. To make board policies
    b. To ensure federal laws are followed
    c. To ensure safe care is given at the lowest cost
    d. All of the above

15. …………….. manages the agency
    a. Board of directors
    b. Administrators
    c. Department directors
    d. Health team head

16. …………leads the health team
    a. Department heads
    b. Department directors
    c. Registered nurse
    d. Administrator

17. All of the following are members of the health team EXCEPT
    a. Clerk

b. Social worker

c. Administrator

d. Activities director

18. .... Is responsible for all nursing care and for the actions of nursing staff during the shift

   a. Charge nurse

   b. Administrators

   c. Head of department

   d. Board of trustees

19. Which of the following is a duty of the registered nurse?

   a. Assess nursing care

   b. Develop care plan

   c. Evaluate care plan

   d. All of the above

20. .... plans and provides care with the health team, does physical exams and health assessment.

   a. Physician

   b. Nurse practitioner

   c. Nursing assistant

   d. Physical therapist

21. .... Is also known as the primary nurse

   a. Nursing assistant

   b. Registered nurse

   c. Licensed vocational nurse

   d. Licensed practical nurse

22. .... Is when services are moved from the departments to the bedside

   a. Patient focused care

   b. Functional nursing

   c. Team nursing

   d. Case management

23. Part B of Medicare pays which of the following expenses?

   a. Hospice expenses

   b. SNF expenses

   c. Doctor's services

   d. All of the above

24. Under the Medicare, ... Is voluntary

   a. Part A

   b. Part B

   c. Part C

   d. None of the above

25. Which of the following does low income earners usually qualify for

   a. Private insurance

   b. Medicaid

   c. Medicare

   d. Group insurance

26. In prospective payment systems .... are used for rehabilitation centers

a. Case mix groups

b. Resource utilization groups

c. Medicare severity adjusted diagnosis related groups

d. Medicaid

27. Which of the following is a type of managed care

   a. Private insurance

   b. Health maintenance organization

   c. Medicare

   d. Group insurance

28. Which of the following can be done if an agency has a deficiency?

   a. Agency can be fined

   b. Agency can lose its license

   c. Agency can lose accreditation

   d. All of the above

29. Surveys are carried out in other to …………

   a. Fine the agency

   b. Ensure different types of care are given

   c. Ensure the agency meets the set standard

   d. Find deficiencies

30. In meeting the set standards you must …………

   a. Provide quality care

   b. Have a good work ethic

   c. Conduct yourself in a professional manner

   d. All of the above

Section 2

The person's right

1. Which of the following explains the person's right and expectations during hospital stays
   a. The Omnibus Budget Reconciliation Act
   b. The Patient Care Partnership: Understanding Expectations Right And Responsibilities
   c. National States Board of Nursing
   d. Health Insurance Portability and Accountability Act Of 1996

2. ………… is someone who supports or promotes the needs and interest of another person
   a. Ombudsman
   b. Representative
   c. Guardian
   d. Nursing centers

3. A representative can be the patient's …………
   a. Partner
   b. Adult child
   c. Court appointed guardian
   d. All of the above

4. A patient has which of the following rights?
   a. Right to information
   b. Right to refuse treatment
   c. Right to personal privacy
   d. All of the above

5. All of the following information may be shared with the patient EXCEPT?
   a. Medical records
   b. Financial records
   c. Doctor's home address
   d. Patient's Health condition

6. In a case of refusal of treatment, the center can do which of the following?
   a. Treat the person still
   b. Offer other treatment options
   c. Send the person back home immediately
   d. All of the above

7. Which of the following must be provided by the health center?
   a. Private rooms
   b. Chapels
   c. Meeting rooms
   d. All of the above

8. All of the following choices can be made by the patient EXCEPT
   A. The type drugs to use
   B. Their doctors
   C. When to get up from bed
   D. What to wear

9. When a grievance is made, the center should do which of the following?
    a. Punish the person for voicing out
    b. Promptly try to correct it
    c. Restrain residents from voicing out
    d. Keep the complaint unresolved until there is confirmation
10. A resident has which of the following rights?
    a. Right to keep and use personal items
    b. Right to be free from abuse
    c. Right to form and take part in resident groups
    d. All of the above
11. Which of the following should be done in a case where you have to inspect a resident's closet
    a. Inspect the closet immediately
    b. Have a co-worker and the resident witness the inspection
    c. Tell the administrator to inspect it by himself
    d. All of the above
12. A center may not employ which of the following persons
    a. A person above 50 years
    b. A male below 22 years
    c. A person found guilty of abusing others by the court
    d. A former resident
13. Which of the following is a form of involuntary seclusion?
    a. Separating the person from others against his or he will
    b. Keeping the person to a certain area
    c. Keeping the person away from his or her room without consent
    d. All of the above
14. .... Reliefs caregivers of daily care for a short time
    a. Respite care
    b. Hospitals
    c. Assisted living residence
    d. Adult day care
15. The older American Act is a ....
    a. State law
    b. Nursing center policy
    c. Federal law
    d. Association of Nursing Act

Section 3
The Nursing assistant

1. Which of the following is a function of the state nurse practice act?
   a. Defines RN and LPN/LVN and their scope of practice
   b. Describes education and licensing requirement for RN and LPN/LVN
   c. Protects the public from person's practicing nursing without a license
   d. All of the above
2. The law can do which of the following to a nursing license?
   a. Deny
   b. Revoke
   c. Suspend
   d. All of the above
3. Which of the following is the ultimate guide that can be used to decide what the nursing assistant can do
   a. States nurse practice Act
   b. Federal nurse practice Act
   c. Center policy
   d. Job description
4. The OBRA requires at least …….. hours of instruction
   a. 20
   b. 40
   c. 75
   d. 100
5. OBRA allows how many attempts to successfully complete evaluation?
   a. 2
   b. 3
   c. 4
   d. 5
6. Which of the following can cause you to lose your certification?
   a. Substance abuse
   b. Giving unsafe care
   c. Violating professional boundaries
   d. All of the above
7. …………. Is a nursing care or a nursing function that can be delegated to nursing assistants when it does not require an RN's professional knowledge
   a. Nursing task
   b. Nursing work
   c. Nursing job
   d. Nursing judgement
8. Which of the following is a job role of a nursing assistant?
   a. Administering drugs

b. Taking phone orders from the doctor

c. Report changes in the persons condition to the nurse

d. Insert tubes into body opening as directed

9. The nursing assistant reports to the ....
   a. Doctor
   b. Nurse
   c. Administrator
   d. All of the above

10. Which of the following should be understood before accepting a job?
    a. Your job descriptions
    b. The ethical and legal aspect of your job
    c. The things you should never do
    d. All of the above

11. .... can delegate tasks to LPN/LVN
    a. RN
    b. Nursing assistant
    c. Doctor
    d. All of the above

12. Which of the following staff cannot delegate?
    a. RN
    b. LPN
    c. Nursing assistant
    d. LVN

13. Before accepting a delegated task which of the following questions should be asked?
    a. Does the state allow you to perform the task
    b. Is it in your job description
    c. Were you trained to do the task
    d. All of the above

14. Which of the following is part of the five rights of delegation?
    a. The right supervision
    b. The right time
    c. The right feedback
    d. The right evaluation

15. You may refuse a task if ....
    a. You don't like it
    b. You don't feel like doing it
    c. You don't know how to use the supplies or equipment
    d. It's time consuming

16. .... is a brief act or behavior outside of the helpful zone
    a. Boundary violation
    b. Boundary crossing
    c. Boundary jumping
    d. Boundary overstepping

17. .... is an act or behavior that meets your needs not the person's need

a. Boundary crossing
b. Boundary jumping
c. Boundary violation
d. Boundary overstepping

18. Which of the following is an example of boundary crossing?
    a. Hugging a crying patient
    b. Abuse
    c. Giving a lot of information about yourself
    d. Keeping secrets with the person

19. Which of the following should be avoided?
    a. Making sexual comments or jokes
    b. Helping the patients with financing
    c. Giving gifts to patients
    d. All of the above

20. Which of the following is a sign of boundary violation?
    a. Spending free time with the person
    b. Flirting with the person
    c. Giving more attention at the expense of other patients
    d. All of the above

21. ……….. is a wrong committed against a person or the person's property
    a. Fraud
    b. Torts
    c. Defamation
    d. Assault

22. Which of the following is an unintentional tort?
    a. Assault
    b. Fraud
    c. Negligence
    d. Battery

23. Preventing a person from leaving the agency is ……….
    a. Invasion of privacy
    b. False imprisonment
    c. Assault
    d. Battery

24. Which of the following is an example of battery?
    a. Touching the person without consent
    b. Giving wrong information
    c. Restraining the person
    d. Threatening to restrain a person

25. ………… is the willful infliction of injury on the patient
    a. Assault
    b. Battery
    c. Abuse
    d. All of the above

26. Which of the following is a sign of self-neglect?
    a. Failing to take needed drugs
    b. Failing to answer call lights
    c. Leaving the person ling in urine
    d. Keeping the persons alone in their room
27. Which of the following is a form of abuse?
    a. Physical abuse
    b. Neglect
    c. Sexual abuse
    d. All of the above
28. All of the following is an example of physical abuse EXCEPT
    a. Hair pulling
    b. Threatening
    c. Depriving the person of basic needs
    d. Whipping
29. Which of the following is a sign of elder abuse?
    a. Depression
    b. Sudden changes in finances
    c. Unexplained withdrawal
    d. All of the above
30. …………abuse occur in relationships
    a. Domestic abuse
    b. Malpractice
    c. Negligence
    d. False imprisonment

Section 4

Work ethics

1. ....involves following laws, being ethical and having the skills to do your work
   a. Professionalism
   b. Team work
   c. Work ethics
   d. All of the above
2. Most adults need .... hours of sleep daily
   a. 5
   b. 8
   c. 10
   d. 12
3. All of the following should be done to maintain hygiene EXCEPT
   a. Use perfumes
   b. Bathe daily
   c. Brush your teeth upon awakening, before and after meal and at bed time
   d. Keep finger nails clean
4. Which of the following should be worn while on duty?
   a. Open toe shoes
   b. Bright colored undergarments
   c. Wristwatch with a second hand
   d. Pierced eyebrows
5. Jobs can be found in which of the following places?
   a. Newspaper ads
   b. Phone book yellow pages
   c. The internet
   d. All of the above
6. Having concern for the person and helping to make the person's life happier is known as being ....
   a. Empathetic
   b. Caring
   c. Trustworthy
   d. Courteous
7. Which of the following qualities is characterized by being gentle and kind towards patient?
   a. Honest
   b. Self-aware
   c. Considerate
   d. Empathetic
8. Which of the following is a trait of good work ethics?
   a. Being cooperative
   b. Being respectful
   c. Being courteous
   d. All of the above

9. To be .... means to accurately report the care given, your observations and any errors
    a. Trustworthy
    b. Honest
    c. Cooperative
    d. Self-aware
10. Which of the following should be done when attending an interview?
    a. Turn off your phone
    b. Be polite
    c. Do not chew gum
    d. All of the above
11. A .... Is a staff member who guides another staff member
    a. Supervisor
    b. Preceptor
    c. Manager
    d. Leader
12. The objective of the orientation program is to ....
    a. Help you feel comfortable in the setting and your role
    b. Help you get to work on time
    c. Help you to be cheerful and friendly
    d. All of the above
13. Which of the following will help you avoid being fired?
    a. Making proper arrangement for your child
    b. Coming late sometimes
    c. Not staying the entire shift
    d. Being absent from your shift
14. Making or writing false statement about another person is ....
    a. Gossip
    b. Fraud
    c. Defamation
    d. Negligence
15. Which of the following is a form of gossip
    a. Talking about patients at home
    b. Making comments that you do not know whether is true about a co-worker
    c. Talking about coworkers on social media
    d. All of the above
16. ....evades a person's privacy
    a. Eavesdropping
    b. Gossiping
    c. Arguing
    d. Lying
17. Which of the following are common courtesies that should be displayed?
    a. Addressing others by Miss, Mrs.,Mr., as appropriate
    b. Saying thank you whenever someone does something for you
    c. Saying am sorry when you make a mistake

d. All of the above

18. Which of the following should be done while at work?
    a. Checking text messages
    b. Making phone calls during breaks
    c. Borrowing money from co-workers
    d. Discussing personal problems

19. Which of the following should be done when you make mistakes?
    a. Blame others
    b. Make excuses
    c. Do not admit your mistakes
    d. Learn from your mistakes

20. Priority setting helps to determine which of the following?
    a. The task to be done first
    b. Who has the greatest need
    c. What task to be done when your shift starts
    d. All of the above

21. ……….. is the response or change in the body caused by any emotional, physical, social or economic factor
    a. Stress
    b. Harassment
    c. Abuse
    d. Threat

22. Which of the following is a physical symptom of stress?
    a. Apprehension
    b. Fear
    c. Sweating
    d. Anger

23. Which of the following is a life threatening problem caused by stress
    a. Muscle tension
    b. Ulcer
    c. Sleep problems
    d. Stomach upset

24. Which of the following can be used to cope with stress?
    a. Exercising regularly
    b. Eating healthy
    c. Getting enough rest
    d. All of the above

25. …… means to trouble or torment a person by one's behavior or comment
    a. Harassment
    b. Defamation
    c. Libel
    d. Battery

Section 5

Communicating with the health team

1. When communicating which of the following should be avoided?
    a. Using words with more than one meaning
    b. Familiar words
    c. Brief and concise words
    d. Giving Facts
2. The ….. is the legal account of a person's condition and response to treatment and care
    a. Nurses report
    b. Output and input report
    c. Medical report
    d. Activities of daily flow sheet
3. Which of the following can be included in the medical chart?
    a. Health history
    b. Admission information
    c. Progress notes
    d. All of the above
4. Which of the following includes the person's identification information?
    a. Nurses note
    b. Progress notes
    c. Admission information
    d. Health history
5. Which of the following is used to record care measures, observations and measurements made daily?
    a. Flow sheets
    b. Health history
    c. Admission information
    d. Medication plan
6. Which of the following information is included in the daily living flow sheet
    a. Bowel movement
    b. Doctor's visit
    c. Weight
    d. All of the above
7. …………. Is used to record current and past illnesses, signs and symptoms, allergies and drugs
    a. Progress notes
    b. Health history
    c. Nurses note
    d. Daily living flow sheet
8. ……….. provides a quick, easy reference to the person's drugs, treatments, diagnosis, care measures, equipment and special needs
    a. Medical record
    b. Observation report
    c. Kardex

    d.   Medical chart

9. The nursing process has ……. Steps
   a. 2
   b. 3
   c. 4
   d. 5

10. ……………. involves collecting information about the person
    a. Investigation
    b. Assessment
    c. Diagnosis
    d. Review

11. Observation is done by ………..
    a. Listening to the person breathe
    b. Seeing how the person walks
    c. Touching the person's skin
    d. All of the above

12. …………. assess the person's body system and mental status
    a. The RN
    b. The nursing assistant
    c. The LVN
    d. The LPN

13. Which of the following is a subjective data?
    a. Flushed skin
    b. Dry skin
    c. Nausea
    d. Wounded body part

14. Which of the following is a nursing diagnosis?
    a. Cancer
    b. Diarrhea
    c. Stroke
    d. Heart attack

15. Which of the following observations must be reported at once?
    a. Vomiting
    b. Bleeding
    c. Dizziness
    d. All of the above

16. Which of the following is contained in a care plan?
    a. Nursing diagnosis
    b. Family health history
    c. Identification information
    d. Vital signs

17. OBRA requires which of the following?
    a. Nursing care plan
    b. Comprehensive care plan

c. Nursing diagnosis

d. Care conference

18. Which of the following is used to communicate delegated measures and task?

    a. Nursing care plan

    b. Delegation schedule

    c. Assignment sheets

    d. Kardex

19. ……… is the oral account of care and observation

    a. Reporting

    b. Recording

    c. Kardex

    d. Implementation

20. Which of the following is included in the end of the shift report?

    a. The care given

    b. The person's current condition

    c. Likely changes in the person's condition

    d. All of the above

21. Which of the following should be done when recording and reporting observations?

    a. Use ditto marks when needed with explanations

    b. Chart a procedure before the procedure is completed

    c. Record in a logical manner

    d. Use correction fluid in case of mistake

22. The ………… is the word element that contains the basic meaning of the word

    a. Root

    b. Prefixes

    c. Suffixes

    d. Stem

23. Nephitis means which of the following?

    a. Difficulty breathing

    b. Inflammation of the kidney

    c. Removal of breast

    d. Inflammation of the liver

24. Endocarditis means which of the following?

    a. Inflammation of the lungs

    b. Inflammation of the inner part of the heart

    c. Inflammation of the kidney

    d. Inflammation of the liver

25. Which of the following is used to describe the front of the body or body part

    a. Anterior

    b. Medial

    c. Proximal

    d. Frontal

26. Which of the following direction term is used to describe the part nearest to the center or from the point of attachment

a. Distal

b. Proximal

c. Lateral

d. Medial

27. Which of the following is a benefit of using computers for recording data?

    a. It is faster

    b. It saves time

    c. Reduces error

    d. All of the above

28. Which of the following should be observed when using computers?

    a. Position the screen towards the hallway

    b. Use e-mail for information or messages that require immediate reporting

    c. Do not write down your username and password

    d. Use emails for to report confidential information

29. Which of the following should be observed when answering a phone call?

    a. End the conversation politely

    b. Return to a caller on hold within 30 seconds

    c. Do not answer the phone in a rushed or hasty manner

    d. All of the above

30. Which of the following violates the Health insurance portability and accountability act of 1996?

    a. Leaving assignment sheets lying around

    b. Using the agency's computer for personal use

    c. Using another person username and password

    d. All of the above

Section 6

Understanding the person

1. Which of the following persons is the most important in the agency?
    a. Patient
    b. Doctor
    c. Nurse
    d. Administrator
2. Which of the following way should patients be addressed?
    a. Their room numbers
    b. Their titles and last name
    c. Grandpa
    d. Their first names without permission
3. Which of the following is a physical need?
    a. Food
    b. Oxygen
    c. Water
    d. All of the above
4. Which of the following is the highest level of the Maslow's hierarchy of needs?
    a. Physical
    b. Love and belonging
    c. Self-actualization
    d. Self esteem
5. Which of the following is the lowest need?
    a. Safe and security
    b. Physical needs
    c. Love and belonging
    d. Self esteem
6. Among the Mexican Americans which of the following illness is caused by exposure to hot conditions?
    a. Constipation
    b. Joint pain
    c. Stomach cramp
    d. All of the above
7. Among the Mexican Americans which of the following illness is caused by exposure to cold conditions?
    a. Constipation
    b. Earache
    c. Sore throat
    d. Fever
8. Which of the following behavior can result from being disabled?
    a. Anger
    b. Withdrawal
    c. Self-centered behavior

    d. All of the above

9. Which of the following shows self-centeredness person?
    a. Becoming impatient if needs are not met
    b. Making inappropriate sexual remarks
    c. Being critical of others
    d. Masturbating in public

10. Which of the following is a sign of anger?
    a. Red face
    b. Rapid speech
    c. Silence
    d. All of the above

11. Which of the following should be observed when communicating with a patient with dementia?
    a. Talk to the person like a baby
    b. Use simple words
    c. Use medical terms as needed
    d. Give lengthy explanations

12. When using verbal communication which of the following should be avoided?
    a. Use of slangs
    b. Shouting and mumbling
    c. Speaking slowly
    d. Using vulgar words

13. In an American, a constant stare with no movement in face muscles shows which of the following?
    a. Coldness
    b. Fear
    c. Tiredness
    d. Embarrassment

14. When using touch, ...
    a. It shouldn't be rough
    b. It shouldn't be hurried
    c. It shouldn't be sexual
    d. All of the above

15. When listening to a person, ...
    a. Hug the person
    b. Face the person
    c. Sit back with your hands crossed
    d. All of the above

16. In the American culture eye contact means which of the following?
    a. Lack of interest
    b. Invasion of privacy
    c. Honesty
    d. Embarrassment

17. Which of the following is a communication barrier?
    a. Unfamiliar language

b. Cultural differences

c. Failure to listen

d. All of the above

18. Which of the following should be avoided when communicating?

    a. Talking too much

    b. Pat answers

    c. Listening attentively

    d. Changing the subject

19. Which of the following is true about a person who is comatose?

    a. He cannot respond to others

    b. He is conscious

    c. He cannot hear

    d. All of the above

20. Bariatric persons are at risk of which of the following problems?

    a. Stoke

    b. Cancer

    c. Diabetes

    d. All of the above

Section 7

Body structure and function

1. The human body is in a steady state of …………
   a. Homeostasis
   b. Psychostasis
   c. Metabolism
   d. Cytoplasm
2. The basic unit of body structure is the ……….
   a. Organ
   b. Cell
   c. Tissue
   d. Nucleus
3. ………….. is the control center of the cell
   a. Cytoplasm
   b. Cell membrane
   c. Nucleus
   d. Protoplasm
4. Which of the following is a function of the nucleus?
   a. It directs the cell's activities
   b. It surrounds the nucleus
   c. It encloses the cell
   d. All of the above
5. Which of the following is true about the protoplasm?
   a. It means living substances
   b. It's a semi liquid substances
   c. It's similar to an egg white
   d. All of the above
6. Each cells has ………… chromosomes
   a. 46
   b. 40
   c. 36
   d. 30
7. Chromosomes contains …………
   a. Cytoplasm
   b. Protoplasm
   c. Genes
   d. Mitosis
8. Which of the following controls cell reproductions?
   a. Hormones
   b. Nucleus
   c. Chromosomes
   d. Genes
9. Which of the following controls trait children inherit from their parent?

a. Nucleus

b. Genes

c. Chromosomes

d. Hormones

10. The process of cell division is called ....

a. Mitosis

b. Cytosis

c. Ketosis

d. Cell division

11. During mitosis the 46 chromosomes arrange themselves in .... Pairs

a. 15

b. 20

c. 23

d. 30

12. Groups of cells with similar function functions combine to form?

a. Tissues

b. Chromosomes

c. Organs

d. System

13. Which of the following is a function of the epithelial tissue?

a. It connects other tissues

b. It covers internal and external body surfaces

c. It lets the body move

d. All of the above

14. Which of the following tissue receives and carries impulses to the brain and back to the body?

a. Connective tissue

b. Epithelial tissue

c. Nerve tissue

d. Muscle tissue

15. Which of the following tissue stretches and contract to let the body move?

a. Nerve tissue

b. Muscle tissue

c. Connective tissue

d. Epithelial tissue

16. Groups of tissue with the same function form ....

a. Organs

b. Cells

c. Systems

d. None of the above

17. The .... is the largest system

a. Skeletal system

b. Muscular system

c. Integumentary system

d. Nervous system

18. There are .... skin layers
    a. 2
    b. 3
    c. 4
    d. 5

19. .... Gives the skin its color
    a. Melanin
    b. Pigment
    c. Dermis
    d. Sudoriferous

20. Which of the following is true about the epidermis?
    a. It is made up of connective tissue
    b. It is supported by subcutaneous tissue
    c. It houses the hair roots
    d. All of the above

21. Which of the following is a function of the skin?
    a. It protects the inside of the body
    b. It prevents microorganisms from entering the body
    c. It protects organ from injury
    d. All of the above

22. Which of the following is true about the dermis?
    a. It is located in the outer layer of the skin
    b. It has living and dead cells
    c. It is made up of connective tissue
    d. All of the above

23. The human body has .... Bones
    a. 200
    b. 206
    c. 109
    d. 102

24. Which of the following is true about long bones?
    a. They bear the body weight
    b. They protect the organs
    c. They allow skill and ease in movement
    d. All of the above

25. .... are the vertebrae in the spinal column
    a. Flat bones
    b. Short bones
    c. Irregular bones
    d. Long bones

26. .... Is needed for bone formation and strength
    a. Magnesium
    b. Phosphorus
    c. Zinc

d. Sodium

27. Blood cells are formed in the ....
    a. Periosteum
    b. Bone marrow
    c. Sebaceous glands
    d. Sudoriferous glands

28. Which of the following is a cushion in the joint that ensures the bone ends do not rub together?
    a. Synovial membrane
    b. Synovial fluid
    c. Periosteum
    d. Ligament

29. Which of the following joints allow movement in all directions?
    a. Hinge joint
    b. Pivot joint
    c. Ball and socket joint
    d. Immovable joints

30. The human body has more than .... Muscles
    a. 500
    b. 1000
    c. 1500
    d. 2000

31. .... Muscles can be consciously controlled
    a. Involuntary
    b. Cardiac muscle
    c. Sphincters
    d. Voluntary

32. Which of the following is a function of the muscles?
    a. It helps in body movement
    b. It helps maintain body posture
    c. It helps in the production of body heat
    d. All of the above

33. .... are circular bands of muscle fibers
    a. Tendon
    b. Sphincters
    c. Achilles
    d. None of the above

34. Which of the following is an opening from the stomach to the small intestine?
    a. Pyloric sphincter
    b. Anal sphincter
    c. Urethral sphincter
    d. Digestive sphincter

35. A .... Is anything that excites or causes a body part to function
    a. Reflex
    b. Stimulus

c. Impulse

d. Fibers

36. Which of the following is a major part of the brain?

a. Cerebrum

b. Cerebellum

c. Brainstem

d. All of the above

37. Which of the following is the largest part of the brain?

a. Brainstem

b. Cerebrum

c. Midbrains

d. Pons

38. Which of the following is controlled by the cerebral cortex?

a. Speech

b. Breathing

c. Swallowing

d. Blood vessel size

39. Which of the following regulates and coordinates body movement?

a. Spinal cord

b. Medulla

c. Cerebrum

d. Cerebellum

40. The spinal cord is about ……… long

a. 5

b. 7

c. 17

d. 24

41. The brain and spinal cord is covered by connectives tissue called …….

a. Meninges

b. Arachnoid

c. Cerebrospinal fluid

d. Spinal nerves

42. The peripheral nervous system has ……. Pairs of cranial nerves

a. 5

b. 10

c. 12

d. 15

43. Which of the following nervous system speeds up body functions?

a. Parasympathetic nervous systems

b. Systematic nervous systems

c. Spinal nervous systems

d. None of the above

44. Which of the following is the outer layer of the eye?

a. Choroid

b. Retina

c. Sclera

d. Iris

45. The .... Separates the cornea from the lens

    a. Aqueous humor

    b. Vitreous humor

    c. Aqueous chamber

    d. Sclera

46. The .... is the second layer of the eye

    a. Choroid

    b. Vitreous humor

    c. Optic nerve

    d. Retina

47. The external ear is called ....

    a. Cerumen

    b. Pinna

    c. Malleus

    d. Ossicles

48. Glands in the auditory canal secretes a waxy substance called ....

    a. Auricle

    b. Pinna

    c. Cerumen

    d. Aqueous humor

49. The ossicles does which of the following?

    a. Amplify sounds received from the eardrum

    b. Separates middle and external ear

    c. Guides sound waves

    d. All of the above

50. .... is the ossicle that looks like an anvil

    a. Malleus

    b. Incus

    c. Stapes

    d. Eustachian tube

51. The malleus looks like ....

    a. Stirrup

    b. Hammer

    c. Anvil

    d. Snail shell

52. The inner ear consists of ....

    a. Cochlea

    b. Temporal bone

    c. Lobe

    d. Tympanic membrane

53. Which of the following is a function of the circulatory systems

a. Blood remove waste products from cells
b. Blood transport the gases of respiration
c. Blood helps regulate body temperature
d. All of the above

54. Which of the following gives blood its red color?
    a. Hemoglobin
    b. Plasma
    c. Platelets
    d. Carbon dioxide

55. The body has about .... Red Blood Cells
    a. 25 billion
    b. 250 billion
    c. 25 trillion
    d. 250 trillion

56. Red blood cells (RBCs) live for about ....months
    a. 4
    b. 10
    c. 12
    d. 24

57. Red blood cells (RBCs) are destroyed by the .... as they wear out
    a. Kidney
    b. Liver
    c. Lungs
    d. Intestine bacteria

58. About .... RBCs are produced every seconds
    a. 1 million
    b. 1 billion
    c. 1 trillion
    d. 10 billion

59. ....protects the body against infection
    a. Red blood cells
    b. Plasma
    c. White blood cells
    d. Protein

60. White blood cells live for about ....
    a. 2 days
    b. 9 days
    c. 1 month
    d. 4 months

61. .... Are needed for blood clotting
    a. White blood cells
    b. Red blood cells
    c. Proteins
    d. Platelets

62. A platelet lives for about ....
    a. 4 days
    b. 10 days
    c. 1 month
    d. 3 months
63. The .... is the outer layer of the heart
    a. Myocardium
    b. Endocardium
    c. Pericardium
    d. Atria
64. Which of the following is a characteristics of the endocardium?
    a. It is a thin sac covering the heart
    b. It lines the inner surface of the heart
    c. It covers the outer layer of the heart
    d. It is the muscular part of the heart
65. The heart has .... chambers
    a. 2
    b. 3
    c. 4
    d. 5
66. The right atrium receives blood from ....
    a. Body tissues
    b. The lungs
    c. The veins
    d. All of the above
67. Which of the following is the function of the right ventricle?
    a. Pumps blood to all parts of the body
    b. Receives blood from the lungs
    c. Receive blood from body tissues
    d. Pumps blood to the lungs
68. The valves allow blood flow in ....
    a. 1 direction
    b. 2 direction
    c. 3 direction
    d. Multiple direction
69. There are .... groups of blood vessels
    a. 2
    b. 3
    c. 4
    d. 5
70. ....are very thin blood vessels
    a. Veins
    b. Arteries
    c. Capillaries

d. Arterioles

71. The veins ……………
    a. Return blood from the heart
    b. Carry blood away from the heart
    c. Receives blood from the left ventricle
    d. Picks up waste products from the cell

72. …………empties into the right atrium
    a. Venules
    b. Superior vena cava
    c. Arterioles
    d. Capillaries

73. ………… carries blood from the legs and trunk
    a. Superior vena cava
    b. Inferior vena cava
    c. Arteries
    d. Capillaries

74. Which of the following is a characteristic of the venous blood?
    a. It is bright red
    b. It is rich in oxygen
    c. It is rich in carbon dioxide
    d. All of the above

75. Blood flows through ………….. into the right ventricle
    a. Femoral artery
    b. Tricuspid valve
    c. Aorta
    d. Superior vena cava

76. The …………pumps blood into the lungs to pick up oxygen
    a. Aorta
    b. Left ventricle
    c. Right ventricle
    d. Right atrium

77. The left ventricle ……………
    a. Pumps blood into the lungs
    b. Empties blood into the right ventricle
    c. Picks up waste from the cells
    d. Pumps blood into the aorta

78. Lymph contains …………
    a. Red blood cells
    b. Proteins
    c. Platelets
    d. All of the above

79. Which of the following is a function of the lymphatic system?
    a. Helps maintain fluid balance
    b. Drains excess fluid from the tissues

c. Defends body against infection

d. All of the above

80. Lymph is transported by ………….

a. Lymphatic tissues

b. Lymphatic arteries

c. Lymphatic vessels

d. All of the above

81. The right lymphatic duct collects lymph from the …………..

a. Right hand

b. Lower chest

c. Abdomen

d. Pelvis

82. The thoracic duct empties into a vein on the ………….

a. Right side of the neck

b. Left side of the neck

c. Right side of the chest

d. Lower chest

83. Lymph nodes are shaped like ………….

a. Hammer

b. Beans

c. Mustard

d. Anvil

84. Lymph nodes are found in the ……………

a. Neck

b. Underarm

c. Chest

d. All of the above

85. The lymph nodes filters …….. from the lymph

a. Cancer cells

b. Blood

c. Excess water

d. All of the above

86. The thymus is usually gone by age ………….

a. 40

b. 60

c. 80

d. 120

87. ………. Is the largest structure in the lymphatic system

a. Thymus

b. Spleen

c. Cisterna chyli

d. Thoracic duct

88. …………. destroys old red blood cells

a. Tonsils

b. Cisterna chyli

c. Spleen

d. All of the above

89. Air contains about ……….. oxygen

a. 21%

b. 40%

c. 50%

d. 90%

90. Air enters the nose and passes through the ……………

a. Bronchus

b. Pharynx

c. Epiglottis

d. Alveoli

91. …………prevent food from entering the airway during swallowing

a. Alveoli

b. Nose

c. Larynx

d. Epiglottis

92. Alveoli picks up ………… from the capillaries

a. Carbon dioxide

b. Oxygen

c. Water

d. Waste

93. The lung is filled with …………

a. Alveoli

b. Blood vessels

c. Nerves

d. All of the above

94. The lungs have …………. Lobes

a. 2

b. 3

c. 4

d. 5

95. Each lung is covered by a 2 layered sac called …………

a. Diaphragm

b. Bronchioles

c. Pleura

d. Alveoli

96. Which of the following is a function of pleura?

a. It secretes fluid that prevents layers from rubbing together during exhalation

b. It saves the iron found in hemoglobin when RBCs are destroyed

c. It prevents food from entering the lungs

d. It filters and removes bacteria

97. The digestive system …………………

a. Removes solid waste from the body

b. Removes carbon dioxide from the body

c. Produces white blood cells

d. Transport food within the blood

98. Which of the following is a major part of the alimentary canal

   a. Mouth

   b. Stomach

   c. Pharynx

   d. All of the above

99. Which of the following is an accessory organ?

   a. Large intestine

   b. Liver

   c. Small intestine

   d. All of the above

100.   ....aids in chewing and swallowing

   a. Taste buds

   b. Salivary gland

   c. Tongue

   d. All of the above

101.   Digestion begins in the …………

   a. Mouth

   b. Stomach

   c. Small intestine

   d. Blood

102.   Taste buds on the tongue' surface contains …….

   a. Veins

   b. Nerve endings

   c. Capillaries

   d. Lymph

103.   Which of the following is true about the stomach?

   a. It is a muscular pouch-like sac

   b. It breaks food into smaller particles

   c. It contains gastric juice

   d. All of the above

104.   The small intestine is about ……

   a. 10 inches long

   b. 20 feet long

   c. 20 inches long

   d. 10 feet long

105.   Tiny projections called ……. Line the small intestine

   a. Villi

   b. Jejunum

   c. Ileum

   d. Chyme

106. Most food absorption takes place in the …………..
    a. Large intestine
    b. Stomach
    c. Ileum
    d. Colon
107. The function of the urinary system is to ……….
    a. Remove waste products
    b. Maintain water balance within the body
    c. Maintain electrolyte balance
    d. All of the above
108. ………….. is needed for the proper function of skeletal and cardiac muscles
    a. Sodium
    b. Potassium
    c. Plasma
    d. Protein
109. A pH of …………. Is neutral
    a. 6
    b. 7
    c. 8
    d. 9
110. Each convoluted tubule has a …….. at one end
    a. Glomerulus
    b. Nephrons
    c. Bowman's capsule
    d. Meatus
111. Urine passes from the bladder through the ……..
    a. Urethra
    b. Ureter
    c. Meatus
    d. Collecting tube
112. …………….is needed for the development of male secondary sex characteristic
    a. Testes
    b. Gonads
    c. Testosterone
    d. Sperm cells
113. From the ……………. Sperm travels to the vas deferens
    a. Scrotum
    b. Seminal vesicle
    c. Ejaculatory duct
    d. Epididymis
114. The ……………….stores sperm and produce semen
    a. Seminal vesicle
    b. Vas deferens
    c. Ejaculatory duct

d. Prostate gland

115. Which of the following is true about the cowper's gland?
   a. It produce semen before ejaculation
   b. It produces testosterone
   c. It passes through the prostate glands
   d. All of the above

116. Which of the following is a function of semen?
   a. It cleanses the urethra
   b. It protects the sperm from damage
   c. It provides lubrication for intercourse
   d. All of the above

117. Which of the following is true about the ovaries?
   a. It contains ova
   b. It secretes estrogen
   c. An ovary is on each side of the uterus in the abdominal cavity
   d. All of the above

118. The main part of the uterus is the ....
   a. Cervix
   b. Fundus
   c. Endometrium
   d. Fallopian tube

119. .... is a small organ composed of erectile tissue
   a. Labia majora
   b. Mons pubis
   c. Clitoris
   d. Bartholin's glands

120. The external female genitalia are called the ....
   a. Vagina
   b. Hymen
   c. Vulva
   d. Clitoris

121. .... is the process in which the lining of the uterus breaks up and is discharged from the body through the vagina
   a. Menstruation
   b. Fertilization
   c. Reproduction
   d. Metabolism

122. Ovulation occurs on or about day .... of the cycle
   a. 10
   b. 14
   c. 20
   d. 22

123. A sperm has .... chromosomes
   a. 10

b. 20

c. 23

d. 30

124.   The endocrine system secretes .... into the bloodstream

a. DNA

b. Hormone

c. Red blood cell

d. Antigens

125.   The .... Gland is called the master gland

a. Pineal gland

b. Thyroid gland

c. Thymus gland

d. Pituitary gland

126.   The anterior pituitary lobe secretes which of the following?

a. Growth hormone

b. Thyroid stimulating hormone

c. Adrenocorticotrophic hormone

d. All of the above

127.   ....prevents the kidneys from excreting excessive amounts of water

a. Antidiuretic hormone

b. Thyroid stimulating hormone

c. Adrenocorticotrophic hormone

d. Oxytocin

128.   Which of the following is a function of oxytocin?

a. It regulates metabolism

b. It regulates growth

c. It causes uterine muscle to contract during child birth

d. It helps the immune system

129.   Parathormone regulates ....

a. Metabolism

b. Calcium use

c. Energy use

d. Growth

130.   ....is important for the development of the immune system

a. Insulin

b. Parathormone

c. Oxytocin

d. Thymosin

131.   The adrenal medulla secretes which of the following?

a. Mineralocorticoids

b. Glucocorticoids

c. Epinephrine

d. Testosterone

132.   ....stimulates the body to quickly produce energy during emergencies

a. Norepinephrine
b. Progesterone
c. Adrenal
d. Mineralocorticoids

133.   Which of the following is a function of Mineralocorticoids?
a. Regulates metabolism of carbohydrates
b. Controls the body's response to stress
c. Regulates the amount of salt and water that is absorbed and lost by the kidney
d. Stimulates the body to quickly produce energy during emergencies

134.   .... Are white blood cells that digest and destroys microorganisms
a. Antibodies
b. Antigens
c. Phagocytes
d. Lymphocytes

135.   The .... produce antibodies that identify and destroy unwanted substances
a. Antigens
b. Lymphocytes
c. Phagocytes
d. Adrenal gland

Section 8

Care of the older person

1. .... is the study of the aging process
   a. Gerontology
   b. Geriatrics
   c. Menopause
   d. None of the above

2. Which of the following is true about aging?
   a. It is normal
   b. It is not a disease
   c. It increases the risk of illness
   d. All of the above

3. At what stage does a person starts to adjust to physical changes?
   a. Adolescence
   b. Young adulthood
   c. Middle adulthood
   d. Late adulthood

4. Which of the following is done at adolescence?
   a. Becoming independent from parents and adults
   b. Choosing a career
   c. Developing moral and ethical behavior
   d. All of the above

5. Which of the following is a social change that occurs with aging?
   a. Reduced income
   b. Severed social relationships
   c. Retirement
   d. All of the above

6. Which of the following physical changes occur with aging?
   a. Wrinkle appearance
   b. Decreased sweating
   c. Dry skin
   d. All of the above

7. Which of the following should be done as aging sets in?
   a. Shampoo hair daily
   b. Bath daily
   c. Engage in exercise
   d. All of the above

8. Which of the following changes occur in the brain with age?
   a. Blood flow to the brain is increased
   b. Recent events are easier to recall than long ago events

    c. Memory is shorter

    d. Sleep periods are longer

9. Which of the following causes fatigue in old people?

    a. Reduced number of red blood cells

    b. Loss of calcium

    c. Decreased secretion from sweat glands

    d. Fewer nerve endings in the skin

10. Which of the following causes dysphagia?

    a. Reduced saliva

    b. Lung tissues are less elastic

    c. Skin loses its elasticity

    d. Red blood cell decrease

11. All of the following changes occur in the digestive system of an old person EXCEPT?

    a. Loss of teeth

    b. Peristalsis increases

    c. Secretion of digestive juices decreases

    d. Fried food may cause indigestion

12. Which of the following foods should aging persons avoid?

    a. Fried food

    b. Fatty food

    c. Dry food

    d. All of the above

13. Which of the following changes may occur in the urinary system of an old person?

    a. Ureters loses elasticity

    b. Bladder size increase

    c. The kidney expands

    d. Blood flow to the kidney is increased

14. Which of the following occur in the reproductive system?

    a. Menopause occurs

    b. Testosterone decreases

    c. Vaginal wall thin

    d. All of the above

15. Which of the following can be done to promote sexuality?

    a. Allow for privacy

    b. Allow grooming routines

    c. Allow married couples to share the same room

    d. All of the above

Section 9

Assisting with safety

1. Which of the following should be reported immediately?
   a. Broken windows
   b. Signs of rodents
   c. Odd smell
   d. All of the above
2. .... is a state of being unaware of one's settings
   a. Coma
   b. Confusion
   c. Disorientation
   d. All of the above
3. A person with impaired vision may not ....
   a. Detect smoke or gas odors
   b. See toys and cords
   c. Hear warning signals
   d. All of the above
4. Which of the following increases the risk of accidents?
   a. Impaired smell
   b. Impaired mobility
   c. Hearing loss
   d. All of the above
5. Which of the following should be done before giving care?
   a. To Identify the person then go and get your supplies
   b. Ask the person to identify him or herself
   c. Use the ID bracelet to identify the person
   d. Use the patient' s face to identify the patient
6. Which of the following can be used to identify the patient?
   a. Bed number
   b. Room number
   c. First names only
   d. ID bracelet
7. All of the following can be done to prevent burns EXCEPT?
   a. Do not pour hot liquid near a person
   b. Do not allow smoking in bed
   c. Keep harmful products in their original label
   d. Don't let the person sleep with heat pad
8. Which of the following is a common cause of burns?
   a. Smoking
   b. Very hot water
   c. Electrical items
   d. All of the above
9. Which of the following can be done to prevent poisoning?

a. Read labels carefully before using a product

b. Clear the airway if the person is choking

c. Stay with the person

d. Do not leave smoking materials at the bedside

10. .... Is when breathing stops from lack of oxygen

    a. Hazard

    b. Poisoning

    c. Suffocation

    d. Choking

11. All of the following can prevent suffocation EXCEPT

    a. Report loose teeth

    b. Encourage the person to keep coughing

    c. Using power strips for care equipment

    d. Use restraints correctly

12. Which of the following can cause choking?

    a. Aspiration of vomitus

    b. Tongue falling back into the airway

    c. Laughing while eating

    d. All of the above

13. Abdominal thrust can be used to relief choking in all of the following persons EXCEPT

    a. 2 year old child

    b. Pregnant woman

    c. Adult over 65

    d. Adult over 18

14. All of the following should be observed for wheelchair and stretcher safety EXCEPT

    a. Check the wheel locks

    b. Check for loose tires

    c. Turnoff the device when done using them

    d. Make sure the castes point forward

15. Which of the following should be done when a warning label is removed or damaged?

    a. Show the container to the nurse

    b. Leave the container

    c. Read the material safety data sheets

    d. Use the content properly

16. Which of the following is a prevention against fire?

    a. Smoke only where allowed to do so

    b. Provide ashtrays into a metal container partially filled

    c. Do not leave cooking unattended to

    d. All of the above

17. Which of the following is needed for a fire?

    a. Cigarette

    b. Spark

    c. Electricity

    d. Oven

18. Which of the following should be done first in case of a fire emergency?
    a. Pull the fire alarm
    b. Use the elevators
    c. Rescue persons in immediate danger
    d. Extinguish the fire
19. Which of the following should be done to prevent elopement?
    a. Monitor and supervise persons at risk
    b. Restrict movement of patients to their rooms
    c. Put an alarm bangle on their feet
    d. Put a tracking device on the patients
20. Which of the following is an example of workplace violence?
    a. Murders
    b. Threats
    c. Kidnapping
    d. All of the above
21. Which of the following should be done when dealing with aggressive patients?
    a. Scold the patients if they try to touch you
    b. Glare at the person to scare him off
    c. Leave the room as soon as you can
    d. Call the police
22. Which of the following is the benefit of risk management?
    a. It helps to prevent accidents
    b. It ensures protection of everyone in the agency
    c. It ensures protection of the agency's property
    d. All of the above
23. Red color coded wristband means ………
    a. Allergy alert
    b. Fall risk
    c. Choking alert
    d. Limb alert
24. Yellow wristbands are used for which of the following?
    a. People with the risk for fall
    b. It warns of food allergy
    c. For a patient with choking risk
    d. As a do not resuscitate order
25. Which of the following is documented in the incident report?
    a. Lost money
    b. Errors in care
    c. Work place violence
    d. All of the above

Section 10

Assisting with fall prevention

1. Which of the following age group is at risk of failing?
   a. 4 to 10
   b. 18 to 25
   c. 25 to 50
   d. 65 and above
2. Falls occurs mostly ………
   a. In the morning
   b. In the bathroom
   c. During lunch
   d. During medication
3. Which of the following patients are at the risk of falls?
   a. Person with disorientation
   b. Persons with depression
   c. Persons with foot problems
   d. All of the above
4. Which of the following will prevent slips?
   a. Slippery bath mat
   b. Floors have glared surface
   c. Use of shower curtains
   d. Skid wax should be used on hardwood
5. Which of the following should be done when water is spilled on the floor
   a. Wipe the spill at once
   b. Floors should be free of clutter
   c. Ensure staffs wear gripped shoes
   d. Ensure power strips are out of the way
6. Which of the following should be done to ensure falls are prevented inside the patient's room?
   a. The bed is at the correct height for the person
   b. Bed and wheelchairs are locked for transfers
   c. Crutches should have non skip tips
   d. All of the above
7. ……….is a device that serves as a guard or barrier along the side of the bed
   a. Bed rail
   b. Hand rail
   c. Grab bars
   d. Gait belts
8. Bed rails should be used for ……….
   a. Stubborn persons
   b. Aggressive persons
   c. Unconscious persons
   d. Elderly persons
9. All of the following should be observed when using bed rails EXCEPT

a. Raise one bed rail if you need to leave the bedside
b. Never leave the person alone when the bed is raised
c. Always lower the bed to a comfortable and safe level
d. All of the above

10. .... Is used to support a person to walk
    a. Wheel chair
    b. Transfer belt
    c. Bed rails
    d. Stretchers

11. Gait belt may be harmful for which of the following patient?
    a. Patient with diabetes
    b. Patient with leg wound
    c. Patient with gastrostomy tube
    d. All of the above

12. Which of the following should be observed when using a transfer belt?
    a. The breast should not be caught under the belt
    b. The belt should be position over the spine
    c. It can be applied on the skin if loosed
    d. It can be applied on the buttocks

13. Which of the following could occur if you try to help a person who is falling?
    a. You could injure yourself
    b. You could injure the patient
    c. Back injuries may occur
    d. All of the above

14. Which of the following should be done after a fall as occurred?
    a. Bring the person up
    b. Call the nurse to check for injuries
    c. Leave the person on the floor
    d. Press the alarm button

15. Which of the following should be done if a patient does not want bed rails?
    a. Remove them
    b. Tell the nurse
    c. Ignore the patient
    d. Administer sedative to keep the patient quiet

Section 11

Restraint alternatives and safe restraint use

1. ...... is any manual method or mechanical device attached to the person's body that he or she cannot remove easily and that restricts freedom of movement to one's body
   a. Physical restraint
   b. Chemical restraint
   c. Psychological restraint
   d. Mental restraint
2. All of the following is true about restraints EXCEPT?
   a. Restraints causes falls
   b. It is used to prevent wandering
   c. Younger persons were more restrained than older persons
   d. Restraints can be used to prevent falls
3. Which of the following is a restraint alternative?
   a. Diversion using TV
   b. Answering call lights promptly
   c. Putting warning devices on beds, chairs and doors
   d. All of the above
4. Which of the following have guidelines for the use of restraints
   a. Center for cancer
   b. Food and drug administration
   c. Medical safety administrators agency
   d. Health insurance act
5. Restraints should be used in which of the following situations?
   a. To control the patient's behavior
   b. To discipline the patient
   c. When necessary to treat medical symptoms
   d. For staff convenience
6. Which of the following is a form of restraint?
   a. Bed rails
   b. Lap-top trays
   c. Tucking in
   d. All of the above
7. The CMS requires the reporting of any death that occurs ....
   a. While the person is in restraint
   b. Within 8 days after a restraint was removed
   c. Within 12 days after the restraint was removed
   d. Within 2 weeks after the restraint was removed
8. Which of the following can occur from the use of restraints?
   a. Diabetes
   b. Infection
   c. Arrhythmias
   d. Kidney disease

9. Which of the following is true about a restrained person
    a. They require more care
    b. They require more supervision
    c. They require more observation
    d. All of the above
10. ………. Gives order for the use of restrain
    a. The RN
    b. Nursing assistant
    c. Doctor
    d. Patients
11. Which of the following should be done before a restraint is applied?
    a. Explain the reason for the restraint to the patient
    b. Other options must have been exploited
    c. Consent must be given before restraint is applied
    d. All of the above
12. All of the following should be observed when restraints are applied EXCEPT?
    a. Follow the manufacturer's instruction
    b. Observe the patients every 12 hours
    c. Protect the person's quality of life
    d. Observe for confusion
13. Which of the following should be done after the restraints have been applied?
    a. Use back cushion when a person is restrained to a chair
    b. Cover the person with a blanket with the restraint underneath in case of cold
    c. Check the person at least every 15minutes
    d. All of the above
14. Which of the following is true about applying restraint?
    a. A person can get suspended and caught between bed rail bars
    b. Straps to prevent sliding should always be around the waist
    c. Criss cross vest or jacket straps should be at the back
    d. All of the above
15. Clothe restraint are applied to the ……….
    a. Ankles
    b. Legs
    c. Thighs
    d. All of the above
16. Leather restraints are applied to the
    a. Hands
    b. Chests
    c. Ankles
    d. Waist
17. Which of the following prevents the use of the finger?
    a. Vest restraints
    b. Wrist restraints
    c. Jacket restraints

    d.   Leather restraints

18. A belt restraint should be used when …………
    a.   There is a risk for pulling out tubes used for life saving treatment
    b.   There is a risk for pulling at devices used to monitor vital signs
    c.   There is a risk for fall
    d.   There is a risk of scratching the skin and causing skin damage

19. Which of the following is a common risk that occurs from the use of vest restraint?
    a.   Strangulation
    b.   Stomach ulcer
    c.   Infection
    d.   All of the above

20. If a mitt restraint is used ensure that ……………
    a.   The patient does not slide forward
    b.   The patient does not ingest the restraints
    c.   The patient does not fall off the chair
    d.   All of the above

21. Which of the following should be observed when applying restraints on the wrist?
    a.   Place the soft part towards the skin
    b.   Secure the restraint tightly
    c.   Ensure that restraint is not loose at all
    d.   Clean the skin with normal saline solution before applying the restraint

22. Which of the following should be noted when applying mitt restraints
    a.   Position the restraint at 90 degrees angle between the wrist and the finger
    b.   Wash the hands in dextrose solution
    c.   Insert the person's hand into the restraints with the palm facing down
    d.   All of the above

23. Which of the following should be noted when applying a belt restraint?
    a.   Position the straps 90 degrees angle between the wheelchair seat and sides
    b.   Secure the restraint to the bed
    c.   Make sure the side seams are under the arms
    d.   Remove wrinkles or creases from the front and back of the restraint

24. Which of the following should be noted when applying vest restraints?
    a.   Criss cross vest straps in the back
    b.   The V part of the vest should cross at the back
    c.   Bring the straps through the slots
    d.   All of the above

25. Which of the following should be noted when using a jacket restraints?
    a.   Assist the person to a sitting position
    b.   Make sure the person is comfortable
    c.   Close the back with the zipper, ties or hook
    d.   All of the above

Section 12

Preventing infection

1. .... is a disease state resulting from the invasion and growth of microbes in the body
   a. Diarrhea
   b. Infection
   c. Nausea
   d. Fever
2. Microbes can be found in the ....
   a. Mouth
   b. Nose
   c. Stomach
   d. All of the above
3. Microbes that are harmful are called ....
   a. Bacteria
   b. Virus
   c. Pathogens
   d. Infections
4. The .... is a place where microbes lives and grow
   a. Reservoir
   b. System
   c. Blood
   d. Portal of dwelling
5. Which of the following is needed for microbes to grow?
   a. Warm environment
   b. Cold environment
   c. Hot environment
   d. None of the above
6. Multidrug resistant organisms are microbes that can resist the effects of ....
   a. Chemotherapy
   b. Antibiotics
   c. Vitamins
   d. Pesticides
7. Methicillin resistant staphylococcus aureus is a bacterium normally found in the ....
   a. Blood
   b. Brain
   c. Nose
   d. Liver
8. Vancomycin resistant Enterococci is a bacterium normally found in the ....
   a. Nose
   b. Intestine
   c. Skin
   d. Ears
9. Vancomycin resistant Enterococci can be transmitted to others through............

a. Sharing of plates
b. Toilet seats
c. Combs
d. Restaurant seats

10. Methicillin resistant staphylococcus aureus can cause …………..
    a. Pneumonia
    b. Urinary tract disease
    c. Pelvic infection
    d. Confusion

11. Vancomycin resistant Enterococci can cause …………
    a. Pneumonia
    b. Serious wound
    c. Pelvic infection
    d. Bloodstream infection

12. Which of the following is a sign of infection?
    a. Fever
    b. Chills
    c. Nausea
    d. All of the above

13. Portal of entry is also the same as the ………….
    a. Carrier
    b. Portal of exit
    c. Reservoir
    d. Source

14. Which of the following are susceptible hosts for infection?
    a. Patients with burns
    b. Chemotherapy patients
    c. Older patients
    d. All of the above

15. Healthcare associated infection is also known as ………….
    a. Nosocomial infection
    b. Socomial infection
    c. Microbial infection
    d. Susceptible infection

16. Which of the following are common sites for Health Associated Infection (HAIs)
    a. Wounds
    b. Respiratory system
    c. Urinary system
    d. All of the above

17. ………… is being free of disease producing microbes
    a. Contamination
    b. Sanitization
    c. Asepsis
    d. Cleaning

18. Medical asepsis is used for which of the following?
    a. Remove pathogens
    b. Prevent pathogens from spreading from one person to another
    c. Destroy pathogens
    d. All of the above
19. Which of the following can be done to prevent the spread of microbes
    a. Wash hands after elimination
    b. Wash hands after changing tampons
    c. Wash fruits before eating
    d. All of the above
20. Which of the following is the easiest and most important way of preventing the spread of infection?
    a. Covering the nose and mouth when coughing
    b. Maintain hand hygiene
    c. Washing cooking utensils
    d. Provide each person with personal care
21. Which of the following should be adhered to?
    a. Wash hands with cold water
    b. Wash hands with water
    c. Use an alcohol based hand rub to practice hand hygiene
    d. Use hot water to wash hands
22. Which of the following should be done when cleaning equipment?
    a. Wear apron
    b. Disinfect the item
    c. Wash the item with water
    d. Work from dirty to clean areas
23. .... is the process of destroying pathogens
    a. Cleaning
    b. Disinfection
    c. Sterilization
    d. Isolation
24. All of the following should be adhered to when using chemical disinfectant EXCEPT?
    a. Use disposable gloves
    b. Read the material safety data sheet
    c. Wear adequate PPE
    d. All of the above
25. .... Is the process of destroying all microbes
    a. Disinfection
    b. Cleaning
    c. Sterilization
    d. Elimination
26. Very high temperatures are used in ....
    a. Cleaning

    b. Sterilization

    c. Disinfection

    d. Elimination

27. Which of the following is a technique used in sterilization?

    a. Radiation

    b. Liquid chemical

    c. Gas chemical

    d. All of the above

28. Which of the following cannot be autoclaved?

    a. Glass

    b. Plastic

    c. Surgical items

    d. Metal

29. Which of the following ways can reservoirs be controlled?

    a. Wash contaminated areas with soap and water

    b. Keep drainage container below the drainage site

    c. Keep tables clean

    d. All of the above

30. Portal of exit can be controlled by …….

    a. Covering your nose and mouth when coughing

    b. Labelling bottles with the person's name

    c. Washing contaminated areas

    d. All of the above

31. Which of the following should be done to control transmissions of microbes?

    a. Shaking lining or equipment slightly

    b. Cleaning from the dirtiest to the cleanest

    c. Clean away from the body

    d. Items picked from the floor should be cleaned before use

32. ………….. are used for all persons whenever care is given

    a. Isolation precaution

    b. Transmission based precaution

    c. Standard precaution

    d. Acceptable precaution

33. There are …….. types of transmission based precautions.

    a. 2

    b. 3

    c. 4

    d. 5

34. Which of the following is a benefit of standard precaution?

    a. It prevent the spread of infection from mucus membrane

    b. It prevent the spread of infection from blood

    c. It prevents the spread of infection from body secretions

    d. All of the above

35. All of the following should be noted when applying standard precautions EXCEPT?

a. Wear gloves when in contact with blood

b. Only re-use gowns when attending to the same person

c. Do not wash gloves for reuse with different persons

d. Remove organic material before disinfection of care equipment

36. A person at risk of transmitting infections to others should be put in a...........

    a. Private room

    b. General room

    c. Emergency room

    d. Surgery room

37. Contact precaution should be used for a patient that is at increase of transferring infection through ....

    a. Respiratory droplets

    b. Airborne route

    c. Contact transmission

    d. All of the above

38. Which of the following is a droplet precaution?

    a. All persons entering the room must wear a TB respirator

    b. Don a mask upon entering the room

    c. The person should be placed in a AIIR

    d. All of the above

39. Which of the following should be removed first when taking off PPE?

    a. Gloves

    b. Googles

    c. Gown

    d. Mask

40. Gloves should be changed in which of the following conditions?

    a. When gloves become contaminated

    b. When moving from contaminated site to clean site

    c. When touching computers

    d. All of the above

41. Which of the following should be adhered to when wearing gowns?

    a. Must cover your neck to your knee

    b. It should cover the arm to elbow

    c. It should be loosed

    d. All of the above

42. A .... Is an item contaminated with blood, body fluids, secretion or excretions

    a. Infectious waste

    b. Bioharzard waste

    c. Contaminated waste

    d. Body waste

43. Which of the following is a bloodborne pathogen

    a. Measles

    b. Chicken pox

    c. Hepatitis B

d. Tuberculosis

44. ………… involves giving a vaccine to produce immunity against an infectious disease
    a. Vaccination
    b. Treatment
    c. Sterilization
    d. Disinfection

45. Occupational safety and health administration requires which of the following practice controls
    a. Never smear or break needle
    b. Do not store food or drinks where blood is kept
    c. Never recap needles by hand
    d. All of the above

Section 13

Body mechanics

1. Body mechanics involves ....
   a. Good posture
   b. Good balance
   c. Using muscles for work
   d. All of the above
2. .... is needed for balance
   a. Base of support
   b. Body alignment
   c. Body mechanics
   d. All of the above
3. The strongest and largest muscles are located in the ....
   a. Brain
   b. Hips
   c. Stomach
   d. Feet
4. Which of the following should be done when lifting heavy objects?
   a. Bend your knees and squat to lift
   b. Bend from the waist to lift
   c. Hold the object away from the body
   d. All of the above
5. All of the following should be avoided EXCEPT?
   a. Unnecessary bending
   b. Sudden or jerky motions
   c. Lifting objects higher than chest level
   d. Using both arms to lift
6. Which of the following is a musculo-skeletal disorder?
   a. Disorder of the brain
   b. Disorder of the joints
   c. Disorder of the liver
   d. Disorder of the lungs
7. Which of the following is a sign and symptom of musculo-skeletal disorder?
   a. Nausea
   b. Dyspnea
   c. Pain
   d. Diarrhea
8. Which of the following is a risk factor for musculo-skeletal disorder?
   a. Old age
   b. Awkward postures
   c. Malnutrition
   d. Depression
9. .... Is the lack of joint mobility caused by abnormal shortening of a muscle

a. Contracture
b. Fracture
c. Seizure
d. Cartilage disorder

10. Which of the following is a benefit of proper positioning?
    a. It makes breathing easier
    b. It promotes comfort and wellbeing
    c. Circulation is promoted
    d. All of the above

11. .... Is a semi sitting position
    a. Supine position
    b. Lateral position
    c. Fowler's position
    d. Prone position

12. .... is the back lying position
    a. Fowler's position
    b. Supine position
    c. Prone position
    d. Lateral position

13. Which of the following is true about the lateral position?
    a. The head of the bed is raised between 45 or 60 degree
    b. The spine is straight up at 90 degree
    c. The upper leg is in front of the lower leg
    d. The person lies on his back

14. Which of the following is true about the prone position?
    a. The person's back is at 45 degree angle with the mattress
    b. The person is in a semi sitting position
    c. Arms are flexed at the elbows with the hands near the head
    d. All of the above

15. .... Helps persons with heart disorders breathe easily
    a. Sim's position
    b. Fowler's position
    c. Prone position
    d. Supine position

Section 14

Assisting with moving and transfers

1. Which of the following guidelines will prevent work related injuries?
   a. Schedule harder task towards the end of your shift
   b. Avoid shoes with worn down soles
   c. Grab the person under the underarm
   d. Let the person hold you around the neck for balance
2. When lifting manually which of the following should guidelines should be followed?
   a. Bend your back
   b. Move the person away from you
   c. Use smooth even movements
   d. All of the above
3. When transporting the person and equipment which of the following guidelines should you adhere to?
   a. Use an upright position
   b. Pull the person gently
   c. Keep the load away from your body
   d. Pull with your whole body gently
4. A person who can bear some weight, sit up and may be able to pivot to transfer is on level ………… of dependence
   a. 2
   b. 3
   c. 4
   d. 5
5. Which of the following is a characteristic of a person on level zero?
   a. The person can walk without help
   b. The person cannot help with transfers
   c. The person is highly involves in the moving or transfer
   d. Stand assist devices may be needed
6. Which of the following is a characteristics of a person on level 4
   a. The staff needs to look after the person
   b. The person needs stand assist devices
   c. The person cannot help at all with the transfer
   d. The person walks without help
7. Which of the following can be done to ease transfer for a patient with dementia?
   a. Use a calm, pleasant voice
   b. Proceed slowly
   c. Divert the person's attention
   d. All of the above
8. ………….. is the rubbing of 1 surface against another
   a. Friction
   b. Shearing
   c. Shredding

d. Smearing

9. Which of the following reduces friction and shearing?
   a. Roll the person
   b. Use a turning sheet
   c. Use a cotton drawsheet
   d. All of the above

10. .... are at great risk of shearing
    a. Neonates
    b. Children
    c. Older persons
    d. Young adults

11. Moving a person in level 4 of dependence require which of the following?
    a. Mechanical lift
    b. One staff
    c. A flat surface
    d. All of the above

12. To move person who weighs 350 pounds will require ....
    a. At least 3 staffs
    b. A friction reducing device
    c. A mechanical lift
    d. All of the above

13. All of the following assistant device can be used to ensure maximum safety EXCEPT?
    a. Disposable under pads
    b. Slide sheet
    c. Drawsheet
    d. Turning pads

14. Which of the following is a benefit of assistant device?
    a. It prevent pain
    b. It prevents injury to the spinal cord
    c. It prevents skin damage
    d. All of the above

15. .... is turning the person as a unit, in alignment, with 1 motion
    a. Dangling
    b. Motioning
    c. Logrolling
    d. Re-positioning

16. During the procedure of logrolling which of the following should be done?
    a. Roll the person away from you
    b. Raise the bed if rails is used
    c. The person may lay on his arm if it is convenient
    d. Place a pillow across his chest

17. Which of the following should be avoided during dangling?
    a. Lowering the bed rail if up
    b. Raising the head of the bed to a sitting position

c. Leaving the person alone

d. Positioning the person in good alignment

18. All of the following information are needed before a transfer is done EXCEPT

   a. Room number

   b. What procedure to use

   c. The person's height and weight

   d. The number of staff needed

19. Which of the following safety measures should be adhered to during transfers?

   a. The person should wear nonskid foot wears

   b. Long gowns and robes should be avoided

   c. Shoe laces should be tightly secured

   d. All of the above

20. Which of the following should be done when transferring a person to a chair?

   a. Lock the wheelchair wheels

   b. Lock the bed wheels

   c. Fan fold top linens to the foot of the bed

   d. All of the above

21. Extended length sling is used for …….

   a. Normal transfers

   b. Persons with extra-large thighs

   c. For amputated persons

   d. For old people

22. ………. Is used with a bariatric lift

   a. Amputee sling

   b. Toilet sling

   c. Bariatric sling

   d. Heavy duty sling

23. Before using the mechanical lift ensure that………..

   a. Only one trained staff may be present

   b. The person's weight must not exceed the lift's capacity

   c. The patient must be lying with the back on the bed

   d. All of the above

24. Using the bathroom for elimination promotes ……….

   a. Dignity

   b. Self esteem

   c. Independence

   d. All of the above

25. Which of the following should be done when transferring a person to and from the toilet?

   a. Close the door for privacy

   b. Help with wiping and flushing

   c. Help the person unfasten clothing

   d. All of the above

Section 15

Assisting with comfort

1. ....affects comfort.
   a. Age
   b. Illness
   c. Activity
   d. All of the above
2. The Center for Medicare & Medicaid Services (CMS) requires that nursing centers maintain a temperature of ....
   a. 50 to 60 degrees
   b. 60 to 70 degrees
   c. 71 to 81 degrees
   d. 81 to 90 degrees
3. Which of the following can be done to reduce odor?
   a. Make sure toilets are flushed
   b. Change wet linens
   c. Keep laundry container close
   d. All of the above
4. According to CMS a comfortable sound level ....
   a. Interferes lightly with a person's hearing
   b. Promotes privacy
   c. Enhances self esteem
   d. Increases life span
5. Which of the following should be done to reduce noise level
   a. Ask others to speak more softly
   b. Have time for light out
   c. Use plastic equipment instead of metal
   d. All of the above
6. ....is usually the sleeping position
   a. High fowler position
   b. Semi fowler position
   c. Flat position
   d. Fowler position
7. In the .... The head of the bed is raised 30 degrees
   a. Semi fowler position
   b. Fowler position
   c. Trendelenburg's position
   d. High fowler position
8. In a reverse Trendelenburg's position the ....
   a. Head of the bed is tilted to 60 degrees
   b. Head of the bed is raised and the foot of the bed is lowered
   c. Head of the bed is lowered the foot raised
   d. Head of the bed is tilted 45 degrees

9. Which of the following is an entrapment zone?
    a. Within the rail
    b. Between the rail and the mattress
    c. Between the split bed rails
    d. All of the above
10. .... holds oral hygiene items
    a. Emesis basin
    b. Wash hand basin
    c. Bedpan
    d. Hygiene pan
11. The call light is connected to ....
    a. The doctor's office
    b. The nurse's station
    c. The reception
    d. The security office
12. Which of the following includes an ambulance stretcher?
    a. Closed bed
    b. Open bed
    c. Surgical bed
    d. All of the above
13. Which of the following should be noted when collecting linen?
    a. Remove all dirty linen together at once
    b. Roll them towards you
    c. Discard the linen in a laundry bag
    d. The side that touch the person should be outside
14. A .... is a small sheet placed over the middle of the bottom sheet
    a. Draw sheet
    b. Absorbtion sheet
    c. Bed protector
    d. Top sheet
15. Which of the following are rules for bedmaking?
    a. Do not use torn or frayed linen
    b. Shake linen subtly to prevent spreads of microbes
    c. Bring extra linen in case of shortage
    d. All of the above
16. The open bed is made for ....
    a. People who arrive through ambulance
    b. Newly admitted person arriving through wheelchair
    c. People returning from surgery
    d. People who are up most of the day
17. The surgical bed is made for persons ....
    a. Who arrive at the agency by through wheelchair
    b. Using portable tubs
    c. Who need muscle stretching

d. Who are on the bed for the most of the day

18. Which of the following can be done to relief pain?
    a. Apply hot water on the area
    b. Provide danceable music to distract the person
    c. Assist with elimination
    d. All of the above

19. Which of the following factors affect reaction to pain
    a. Past experience
    b. Anxiety
    c. Age
    d. All of the above

20. Which of the following promotes sleep
    a. Avoid caffeine and alcoholic drinks
    b. Give a back massage
    c. Provide a bedtime snack
    d. All of the above

21. Protein tryptophan can be found in which of the following?
    a. Milk
    b. Beans
    c. Millet
    d. Butter

22. Exercise should be avoided .... before bedtime
    a. 6 hours
    b. 5 hours
    c. 3 hours
    d. 2 hours

23. .... is a chronic condition in which the person cannot sleep or stay asleep all night
    a. Anosmia
    b. Insomnia
    c. Sleepwalking
    d. Sleep deprivation

24. Which of the following is a form of insomnia?
    a. Cannot fall asleep
    b. Cannot stay asleep
    c. Cannot fall back asleep
    d. All of the above

25. During .... the person is not aware of the event of awakening
    a. Insomnia
    b. Anosmia
    c. Sleep walking
    d. Sleep deprivation

Section 16

Assisting with hygiene

1. Which of the following is the first line of defense against disease?
   a. Blood
   b. Skin
   c. Eyes
   d. Hands
2. Which of the following is a benefit of oral hygiene?
   a. Prevent mouth odors
   b. Increases comfort
   c. Makes food taste better
   d. All of the above
3. Which of the following can cause periodontal disease?
   a. Plague
   b. Malnutrition
   c. Dry mouth
   d. Mouth odor
4. .... is breathing fluid, food, vomitus or an object into the lungs
   a. Choking
   b. Periodontal disease
   c. Aspiration
   d. Supine disease
5. Which of the following can be done to prevent aspiration?
   a. Position the person flat on the bed
   b. Use small amount of fluid
   c. Carefully insert dentures if the person is unconscious
   d. Use your fingers only after wearing gloves
6. Which of the following is a procedure for cleaning dentures?
   a. Use toothpaste and mouthwash to clean the denture
   b. Soak it in hot water to remove microbes
   c. Store the denture in a dry sealed container to prevent infection
   d. Rinse the denture under running water
7. Which of the following is a benefit of bathing?
   a. It cleans the skin
   b. It is relaxing and refreshing
   c. It stimulates circulation
   d. All of the above
8. When bathing a patient ....
   a. Use soap to wash around the eyes and face
   b. Only the genitals should not be exposed
   c. Allow the person perform perineal care
   d. Use hot water to bath the person
9. Which of the following bath options is appropriate for a paralyzed patient?

a. Complete bed bath

b. Partial bath

c. Tub bath

d. Shower

10. The …………. bath is relaxing

a. Shower

b. Tub

c. Complete bed bath

d. Partial

11. A tub bath can last …………

a. 10 minutes

b. 30 minutes

c. 45 minutes

d. 60 minutes

12. When a patient is bathing ………..

a. Block the drainage

b. Stay in the bathroom

c. Knock before entering

d. All of the above

13. Perineal care is very important for which of the following people

a. Unconscious persons

b. Persons menstruating

c. Paralyzed patients

d. None of the above

14. When giving perineal care which of the following should be adhered to?

a. Clean from the front to the back

b. Report any redness or swelling

c. Use warm water

d. All of the above

15. A decision of whether to shower or to have a tub bath should be made by the………

a. Nurse

b. Patient

c. Nursing care plan

d. Doctor

Section 17

Assisting with grooming

1. Alopecia is signified by ....
   a. Hair loss
   b. Dry scalp
   c. Excessive hair
   d. Infestation with lice
2. .... is excessive body hair
   a. Scabies
   b. Alopecia
   c. Hirsutism
   d. Pediculosis
3. Which of the following can cause alopecia?
   a. Old age
   b. Chemotherapy
   c. Heredity
   d. All of the above
4. ....is the infestation of scalp with lice
   a. Pediculosis capitis
   b. Pediclosis pubis
   c. Pediculosis corporis
   d. Pediculosis crab
5. Lice can be spread through...........
   a. Beds
   b. Towels
   c. Sexual contact
   d. All of the above
6. .... is a skin disorder caused by the female mite
   a. Dandruff
   b. Pediculosis
   c. Scabies
   d. Alopecia
7. Which of the following is a sign of pediculosis?
   a. Itching
   b. Nausea
   c. Vomiting
   d. All of the above
8. .... is the infestation of the pubic hair with lice
   a. Pediculosis capitis
   b. Pediclosis pubis
   c. Pediculosis corporis
   d. Pediculosis crab
9. Which of the following is a common site of scabies?

a. Breast

b. Buttocks

c. Underarms

d. All of the above

10. Which of the following is a sign of scabies?

a. Rash

b. Dyspnea

c. Nausea

d. Fever

11. Which of the following should be done if a patient has scabies?

a. Clean the room

b. Wash linens with hot water

c. Maintain hand hygiene

d. All of the above

12. A person who has limited range of motions in her head should be shampooed...........

a. On a stretcher

b. At the sink

c. In bed

d. All of the above

13. Which of the following observation should be reported if seen during brushing of hair?

a. Scalp sores

b. Flaking

c. Itching

d. All of the above

14. Which of the following guidelines should be noted when shaving?

a. Use only safety razors

b. Soften the beard before shaving

c. Shave towards the ankles

d. All of the above

15. Safety razors can be used for ....

a. Persons taking anticoagulant drugs

b. Dementia patients

c. Patients with alopecia

d. All of the above

16. Which of the following safety guidelines should be followed when using safety razors?

a. Apply talcum powder before shaving

b. Lather the face with soap

c. Soak the razor in hot water

d. Use disinfectant to clean the razor

17. Feet odor is caused by..........

a. Dirty feet

b. Stubbing on toes

c. Stepping on sharp objects

d. Poor fitted shoes

18. Which of the following causes poor circulation in the feet?
    a. Infections
    b. Injuries
    c. Diabetes
    d. Microbes
19. All of the following should be adhered to when providing nail and foot care EXCEPT?
    a. Trim and clean after soaking or bathing
    b. Use scissors for hard nails
    c. Use nail clippers for fingernails
    d. Apply petroleum jelly to the feet
20. Which of the following is a rule for dressing and undressing?
    a. Provide privacy
    b. Choose appropriate dressing
    c. Remove clothing from the weak side first
    d. Put clothing on the strong side first

Section 18
Assisting with urinary elimination

1. A healthy adult produces about .... of urine a day
    a. 1 pint
    b. 3 pints
    c. 5 pints
    d. 8 pints

2. Which of the following affects urine production?
    a. Age
    b. Body temperature
    c. Drugs used
    d. All of the above

3. ....is known as blood in the urine
    a. Dysuria
    b. Polyuria
    c. Hematuria
    d. Oliguria

4. Oliguria occurs when .... of urine is voided in 24 hours
    a. 400ml
    b. 600ml
    c. 700ml
    d. 800ml

5. .... Is also known as frequent urination at night
    a. Polyuria
    b. Nocturia
    c. Dysuria
    d. Oliguria

6. Dysuria is known as ....
    a. Difficult urination
    b. Inability to urinate
    c. Urinary incontinence
    d. Abnormal urine

7. Fracture pans are used by ....
    a. Persons with cast
    b. Persons with traction
    c. Persons with limited back motion
    d. All of the above

8. Which of the following is a normal color of urine?
    a. Red
    b. Tea
    c. Amber
    d. Yellow

9. .... is the involuntary loss or leakage of urine
    a. Urinary incontinence

b. Urinary infection

c. Urinary frequency

d. Urinary urgency

10. Urine leaks during exercise and certain movement that cause pressure on the bladder is known as

a. Urge incontinence

b. Overflow incontinence

c. Stress incontinence

d. Functional incontinence

11. Which of the following is a cause of reflex incontinence?

a. Nervous system disorders

b. Confusion

c. Immobility

d. Disorientation

12. In .... the person feels like the bladder is not empty

a. Stress incontinence

b. Urge incontinence

c. Overflow incontinence

d. Functional incontinence

13. In functional incontinence the person ....

a. Does not feel the need to void

b. Cannot use the toilet in time

c. Feels like the bladder is not empty

d. Has urine dribbling

14. In ....the person has a combination of stress incontinence and urge incontinence

a. Combined

b. Mixed incontinence

c. Reflex incontinence

d. Functional incontinence

15. .... Refers to temporary or occasional incontinence that is reversed when the cause is treated

a. Transient incontinence

b. Occasional incontinence

c. Temporary incontinence

d. Flexible incontinence

16. Which of the following is a cause of urinary incontinence?

a. Rectal surgery

b. Intestinal surgery

c. Reproductive system surgery

d. All of the above

17. All of the following are true about urinary incontinence EXCEPT

a. Older persons are at risk

b. It is embarrassing

c. It is a normal part of aging

d.   It can cause depression

18. Which of the following precautions can be used to prevent urinary tract infection?
   a.   Keep the perineal area clean and dry
   b.   Promote fluid intake as the nurse directs
   c.   Have the person wear cotton underwear
   d.   All of the above

19. All of the following should be done to manage urinary incontinence EXCEPT
   a.   Assist with elimination before bedtime
   b.   Leave urinals in place to catch urine for men
   c.   Have the person wear easy to remove cloth
   d.   Apply a barrier cream as directed by the nurse

20. Which of the following should be noted when using incontinence products?
   a.   Center the product in the perineal area
   b.   Do not let the plastic backing touch the person's skin
   c.   Position the penis downwards
   d.   All of the above

21. Which of the following is true of catheters
   a.   It is used for weak persons
   b.   It is usually done by nursing assistance
   c.   It can be used to treat incontinence
   d.   It cannot protect wounds from contact with the skin

22. Which of the following guidelines should be followed when using indwelling catheter?
   a.   Tubing should not have kinks
   b.   Attach the drainage bag to the bed rail
   c.   Let the drainage bag rest on a disinfected floor
   d.   All of the above

23. Which of the following will prevent excess catheter movement and friction at the insertion site?
   a.   Secure the catheter to the bed rail
   b.   Secure the catheter to the man's abdomen
   c.   Place the drainage bag close to the bed rail
   d.   Secure the drainage bag on the bed beside the patient

24. Which of the following is a sign and symptom of urinary tract infection?
   a.   Fever
   b.   Blood in the urine
   c.   Chills
   d.   All of the above

25. Leg bags holds less than .... of urine
   a.   200ML
   b.   500ML
   c.   1000ML
   d.   2000ML

26. Standard drainage bags usually holds at least .... of urine
   a.   2000ML

    b. 1000ML

    c. 500ML

    d. 200ML

27. Which of the following is true about drainage systems?

    a. The standard drainage bags fill faster than the leg bags

    b. Infection can occur if microbes enter the drainage system

    c. It should be emptied only at the end of each shift

    d. All of the above

28. Which of the following guidelines should be observed when applying condom catheters?

    a. Do not apply if the penis is red

    b. Act in professional manner

    c. Use only elastic tape

    d. All of the above

29. ………….. Is when voiding is scheduled at regular times to match the person's voiding habits

    a. Catheter clamping

    b. Habit training

    c. Prompted voiding

    d. Bladder rehabilitation

30. During bladder retraining the person needs to ………..

    a. Postpone or delay voiding

    b. Resist or ignore the urge to urinate

    c. Urinate following a schedule

    d. All of the above

Section 19

Assisting with bowel elimination

1. Which of the following factors affect the frequency, consistency, color and odor of stool?
   a. Privacy
   b. Habits
   c. Diet
   d. All of the above
2. Which of the following food aids bowel movement?
   a. Beans
   b. Bread
   c. Potatoes
   d. Chicken
3. Drinking ………….. glasses of water daily promotes normal bowel movement
   a. 2
   b. 3
   c. 4
   d. 8
4. Which of the following should be provided during bowel elimination?
   a. Cover the person for warmth and privacy
   b. Provide perineal care
   c. Warm the bedpan
   d. All of the above
5. ……… is the passage of a hard, dry stool
   a. Flatulence
   b. Constipation
   c. Fecal impaction
   d. Diarrhea
6. …………. Is the prolonged retention and buildup of feces in the rectum?
   a. Fecal impaction
   b. Fecal incontinence
   c. Flatulence
   d. Constipation
7. Which of the following is a cause of constipation?
   a. Enemas
   b. Decreased fluid intake
   c. Suppositories
   d. All of the above
8. Which of the following is a sign or symptoms of fecal impaction?
   a. Fever
   b. Dyspnea
   c. Arrhythmias
   d. Diarrhea
9. Which is true about diarrhea?

a. The person cannot have a bowel movement

b. More water is absorbed from hard feces

c. The need for bowel movement is urgent

d. All of the above

10. Which of the following is a cause of diarrhea?

a. Microbes in foods

b. Contaminated water

c. Infection

d. All of the above

11. Which of the following is a sign and symptom of diarrhea?

a. Loss of appetite

b. Chronic Pain

c. Sepsis

d. Insomnia

12. Which of the following is a cause of fecal incontinence

a. Diarrhea

b. Mental health disorder

c. Aging

d. All of the above

13. Which of the following is a cause of flatulence?

a. A low fiber diet

b. Decreased fluid intake

c. Constipation

d. Drugs

14. A……. is a cone shaped, solid drug that is inserted into a body opening that promotes bowel movement

a. Enemas

b. Suppository

c. Flatus

d. Intestinal peristalsis

15. Which of the following is a function of enemas?

a. To remove feces

b. To gain control of bowel movement

c. To ensure pattern of elimination

d. To prevent fecal incontinence

16. Saline enema contains …………

a. Castile soap

b. Mineral oil

c. Table salt

d. Alcohol

17. For adult soapsuds enema add ……… of castile soap to 500 to 1000ml of tap water

a. 4ML

b. 7ML

c. 9ML

d. 15ML

18. Which of the following guidelines should be adhered to when giving enemas?
    a. Lubricate the enema tip before inserting it
    b. Hold the enema bag 30 inches above the anus
    c. Position the patient in a semi fowler position
    d. All of the above

19. Usually it takes …………to give 750 to 1000ML of enema solution
    a. 1 to 2 minutes
    b. 5 to 6 minutes
    c. 10 to 15 minutes
    d. 30 to 45 minutes

20. Which of the following is a reason for removing a part of the intestine?
    a. Cancer
    b. Bowel disease
    c. Trauma
    d. All of the above

21. ………….. is a surgically created opening between the colon and the abdominal wall
    a. Ostomy
    b. Colostomy
    c. Stomatomy
    d. Ileostomy

22. The more …………. remaining to absorb water, the more solid and formed the stool
    a. Tubing
    b. Colon
    c. Stoma
    d. Enema

23. ………. Is a surgically created opening between the small intestine and the abdominal wall
    a. Ostomy
    b. Stomatony
    c. Ileostomy
    d. Colostomy

24. Which of the following is true about stools?
    a. It irritates the skin
    b. It can cause skin break down
    c. It must not touch the skin
    d. All of the above

25. Which of the following is true?
    a. Wipe the drain of the ostomy pouch before closing
    b. Peristalsis decreases after food
    c. After sleep stomas are more likely to prevent feces
    d. Change ostomy pouches every day

Section 20

Assisting with nutrition and fluids

1. A poor diet and poor eating habit can …………
   a. Increase the risk for disease and infection
   b. Cause healing problems
   c. Increase the risk for accidents and injuries
   d. All of the above
2. Which of the following is a group of nutrient?
   a. Fats
   b. Proteins
   c. Carbohydrates
   d. All of the above
3. 1 gram of carbohydrate is equal to ………..
   a. 9 calories
   b. 6 calories
   c. 4 calories
   d. 2 calories
4. The Unites state department of agriculture recommends that adults do at least which of the following?
   a. 15 minutes each week of vigorous physical activity
   b. 1 hour each of moderate physical activity
   c. 2 days a week of strengthening activities
   d. All of the above
5. Which of the following is an example of vigorous physical activities?
   a. Running and jogging
   b. Golf
   c. Tennis
   d. Dancing
6. Whole grains …………
   a. Have less dietary fiber
   b. Have the entire grain kernel
   c. Have fine texture
   d. All of the above
7. Which of the following is a benefit of grains to the body?
   a. Reduces the risk of kidney stones
   b. It helps for bone and tooth formation
   c. Helps prevent constipation
   d. All of the above
8. Which of the following is in the group of dark green vegetables
   a. Turnips
   b. Bananas
   c. Green peas
   d. Celery

9. Which of the following is a benefit of fruit to the body?
   a. May reduce the risk of bone loss
   b. Contains no cholesterol
   c. It is low in sodium
   d. All of the above
10. Which of the following belongs to the milk group?
    a. Cheese
    b. Cream
    c. Butter
    d. All of the above
11. All of the following contains high cholesterol EXCEPT?
    a. Egg white
    b. Liver
    c. Regular ground beef
    d. Chicken with skin
12. Which of the following is true about oils?
    a. Oils are low in calories
    b. The best oil choice comes from fish and nuts
    c. Oils from plants contain cholesterol
    d. Oils and fat have about 12 calories in each spoon
13. .... is needed for tissue growth
    a. Minerals
    b. Water
    c. Protein
    d. Fat
14. Which of the following is true?
    a. Appetite usually decreases during illness
    b. People with limited income often buy cheaper carbohydrate foods
    c. Nutritional needs increases during illness
    d. All of the above
15. Which of the following is a requirement from omnibus budget reconciliation Act for food served in nursing centers?
    a. Foods should be appetizing
    b. Hot food should be severed hot
    c. Food should be well seasoned
    d. All of the above
16. The body needs no more than .... of sodium day
    a. 5000mg
    b. 4000mg
    c. 2300mg
    d. 1300mg
17. Healthy people secrete or excrete excess sodium in ....
    a. Urine
    b. Sweat

c. Feces

d. All of the above

18. .... causes the body to retain water

a. Calcium

b. Potassium

c. Sodium

d. Chloride

19. Which of the following occurs when there is too much sodium in the body?

a. The person is more energetic

b. The heart works harder

c. Food is not quickly digested

d. All of the above

20. .... are foods liquid at body temperature and leaves small amount of residue usually used after surgery

a. Full liquid

b. Clear liquid

c. Mechanical soft

d. Fiber

21. Which of the following foods should be consumed in case of diarrhea?

a. Yogurt

b. Raw Fruits

c. Raw Vegetables

d. Refined bread

22. Which of the following should be consumed in case of constipation?

a. Butter

b. Refined bread

c. Crackers

d. All of the above

23. .... are foods that are non-irritating and low in roughage, served at moderate temperature without strong spices

a. High fiber

b. Mechanical soft

c. Bland

d. Full liquid

24. Which of the following should be consumed for weight loss?

a. Candy

b. Lean meats

c. Noodles

d. Rice

25. Which of the following should be consumed by a patient with liver disease

a. Cottage cheese

b. Sherbet

c. Fruit

d. All of the above

26. In a diabetes meal plan …………..
    a. The same amount of protein, carbohydrates and fats are eaten in a day
    b. A certain amount of sodium is allowed
    c. Foods high in iron are served
    d. 3000 calories is served daily
27. Which of the following food is high in sodium?
    a. Waffles
    b. Pepperoni
    c. Cheese
    d. All of the above
28. Which of the following should be observed for a patient with diabetes?
    a. Ensure that meals and snacks are taken at regular times
    b. Meals and snacks should be served on time
    c. Always check what was eaten
    d. All of the above
29. …………..means that the food enters the airway
    a. Slow swallow
    b. Unsafe swallow
    c. Dysphagia
    d. None of the above
30. Which of the following is a sign and symptom of dysphagia?
    a. Food comes out from the nose
    b. Nausea
    c. Vomiting
    d. All of the above
31. An adult needs ………… of water daily to survive
    a. 250 ml
    b. 500ml
    c. 1000ml
    d. 1500ml
32. When is non per os is ordered?
    a. To encourage increased fluid intake
    b. Before surgery
    c. To restrict fluid intake
    d. To maintain body balance
33. Which of the following is a common type of dinning program?
    a. Social dinning
    b. Open dinning
    c. Low stimulation dinning
    d. All of the above
34. Which of the following should be adhered to when feeding a person?
    a. Use small forks when feeding
    b. Offer fluids during the meal
    c. Let them hold hot drinks with handle

d. All of the above

35. ....is a feeding tube inserted through the nose into the stomach
    a. Gastrostomy tube
    b. Gavage tube
    c. Naso gastric tube
    d. Gastro intestinal tube

36. Aspiration can occur in which of the following instances?
    a. During insertion of NG tube
    b. During increased pulse rate
    c. During coughing
    d. All of the above

37. Which of the following can be done to prevent regurgitation and aspiration?
    a. Avoid the left side lying position
    b. Maintain the sims position after eating
    c. Position the person in a sims position before eating
    d. All of the above

38. Which of the following is a comfort measure for person's feeding on tubes?
    a. Clean the nose and nostrils every 1 to 2 hours
    b. Re-tape the nose
    c. Secure the tube to the person's garment at the shoulder area
    d. All of the above

39. Which of the following is a sign or symptom of IV therapy complication
    a. Bleeding at the site
    b. Fever
    c. Nausea
    d. All of the above

40. Which of the following functions can nursing assistant perform?
    a. Start IV therapy
    b. Regulate flow rate
    c. Report sign and symptoms
    d. Change IV bags

Section 21

Assisting with assessment

1. Vital signs reflect the function of ……….. body processes
   a. 3
   b. 4
   c. 5
   d. 6
2. Which of the following is a vital sign of body function?
   a. Temperature
   b. Pulse
   c. Respiration
   d. All of the above
3. Which of the following is a benefit of taking measuring vital signs?
   a. To detect changes in normal body function
   b. To know treatment responses
   c. It show signals of life threatening events
   d. All of the above
4. Heat is produced ………….
   a. When taking hot shower
   b. When sitting down
   c. As cells use food for energy
   d. As energy is being consumed
5. Heat is lost through ………..
   a. Saliva
   b. Breathing
   c. Sleep
   d. Crying
6. Body temperature is usually lower in the ………….
   a. Morning
   b. Afternoon
   c. Evening
   d. All of the above
7. Which of the following is a temperature site?
   a. Hand
   b. Mouth
   c. Nose
   d. Thighs
   e. All of the above
8. Oral temperatures should not be taken if the person …………….
   a. Is above 5 years of age
   b. Is unconscious
   c. Has diarrhea
   d. Is confused or agitated

9. Which of the following sites is used in infants?
    a. Oral site
    b. Axillary site
    c. Rectal site
    d. Temporal artery site
10. Axillary site is ....
    a. Less reliable than the other site
    b. Used for infants
    c. Not used for persons under 3
    d. Non invasive
11. Rectal temperature should not be taken if the person ....
    a. Has sore mouth
    b. Has an ear disorder
    c. Has heart disease
    d. Has a convulsive disorder
12. Which of the following is true?
    a. Oral temperatures should not be taken if the person is paralyzed on one side of the body
    b. Rectal sites should not be used if the person has a rectal disorder
    c. Older persons have lower body temperature
    d. All of the above
13. The baseline body temperature for the oral site is ....
    a. 98.6^oF
    b. 99.6^oF
    c. 97.6^oF
    d. 96.6^oF
14. The tympanic membrane thermometer measures body temperature in the ....
    a. Oral site
    b. Rectal site
    c. Tympanic membrane
    d. Forehead
15. ....have a hollow glass tube and a bulb tip
    a. Standard electronic thermometer
    b. Tympanic membrane thermometer
    c. Glass thermometer
    d. Digital thermometer
16. Which of the following measures body temperature at the oral, rectal and axillary sites?
    a. Digital thermometer
    b. Temporal artery thermometer
    c. Tympanic membrane thermometer
    d. All of the above
17. Which of the following thermometer is safe for older persons who are confused?
    a. Standard electronic thermometer
    b. Tympanic membrane thermometer
    c. Glass thermometer

d. All of the above

18. Which of the following is a benefit of using glass thermometers
    a. It is quick to register
    b. It is re-usable
    c. There is low risk of infection
    d. All of the above

19. A pulse is felt every time ....
    a. The nose breathes
    b. The heart beats
    c. We sneeze
    d. We move

20. The .... pulse is used more often
    a. The apical
    b. Femoral
    c. Radial
    d. Popliteal

21. The apical pulse is ....
    a. In the thighs
    b. On the forehead
    c. On the hand
    d. Below the left nipple

22. The temporal pulse in found ....
    a. On the forehead
    b. On the knee
    c. In the arm
    d. In the chest

23. Which of the following guidelines should be followed when using stethoscope?
    a. Wipe the ear pieces and diaphragm with antiseptic wipes before and after use
    b. Ask the person to be silent
    c. Place the diaphragm over the pulse site
    d. All of the above

24. The pulse rate is the number of heartbeats or pulses felt or heard in ....
    a. 1 minute
    b. 2 minute
    c. 30 seconds
    d. 45 seconds

25. Which of the following guidelines should be adhered to when taking pulses?
    a. Place 2 finger tips on the palm
    b. Count the pulse for 2 minutes
    c. Use stethoscope to count apical pulse for one minute
    d. Count the lub as one beat

26. The apical pulse is located.............
    a. Under the nipple
    b. 2 inches to the left of the sternum

c. 2 inches to the right of the heart

d. 3 inches to the right of the heart

27. Which of the following is true about respiration?

   a. Each respiration involves one inhalation only

   b. Each respiration involves exhalation only

   c. The chest rises during inhalation

   d. The chest falls during inhalation

28. The healthy adult has ……. respiration Per minute

   a. 2 to 5

   b. 5 to 10

   c. 12 to 20

   d. 20 to 35

29. To count respiration ……………

   a. Watch the chest rise and fall

   b. Tell the person to breathe in and out

   c. Keep your eyes on the stethoscope

   d. All of the above

30. …………is the amount of force exerted against the walls of an artery by the blood

   a. Pulse

   b. Blood pressure

   c. Temperature

   d. Pain

31. ………..is the period of heart muscle contraction

   a. Diastole

   b. Hypertension

   c. Systole

   d. Blood pressure

32. ………… is the pressure in the arteries when the heart is at rest

   a. Diastolic pressure

   b. Hypertension

   c. Hypotension

   d. Systolic pressure

33. Which of the following is in the range of a systolic pressure?

   a. 60 mm Hg or higher but lower than 80 mm Hg

   b. 140 mm Hg or higher

   c. 120 mm Hg or higher

   d. 90 mm Hg or higher but lower than 120 Hg

34. Which of the following manometer has a round dial and a needle that points to the numbers?

   a. Mercury manometer

   b. Aneroid manometer

   c. Electronic manometer

   d. Mechanical manometer

35. Which of the following should be avoided?

   a. Taking blood pressure on an arm with an IV infusion

b. Taking BP on an arm with an arm crest
c. Taking BP on an arm on the side of breast surgery
d. All of the above

36. If you are not sure of the accuracy of the BP wait .... before you repeat the measurement
    a. 10 seconds
    b. 20 seconds
    c. 30 seconds
    d. 3 minutes

37. .... is felt suddenly from injury, disease or surgery
    a. Acute pain
    b. Chronic pain
    c. Radiating pain
    d. Phantom pain

38. ....continues for a long time or occurs off and on
    a. Chronic pain
    b. Continuous pain
    c. Radiating pain
    d. Acute pain

39. Which of the following is a common cause of chronic pain?
    a. Back pain
    b. Arthritis
    c. Heart attack
    d. Gallbladder

40. .... is felt in a body part that is no longer there
    a. Imaginary pain
    b. Continuous pain
    c. Phantom pain
    d. Frictional pain

41. Which of the following is a sign and symptom of pain?
    a. Nausea
    b. Vomiting
    c. Groaning
    d. All of the above

42. Which of the following should be recorded when reporting the pain of a patient?
    a. Location of the pain
    b. Intensity of the pain
    c. Onset and duration of the pain
    d. All of the above

43. Which of the following should be measured at output?
    a. Ice cream
    b. Pudding
    c. Urine
    d. Gelatin

44. One quart is about ....

a. 30ml
b. 500ml
c. 1000ml
d. 2000ml

45. Which of the following guidelines should be followed when measuring weight and height?
    a. No footwear is worn
    b. The person voids before being weighed
    c. Weigh the person at the same time of the day
    d. All of the above

Section 22

Assisting with specimens

1. All specimens sent to the laboratory require ……….
   a. Requisition slip
   b. Nurse care plan
   c. Kardex
   d. Assignment sheet
2. Which of the following rules should be adhered to when collecting specimens?
   a. Do not touch the inside of the container
   b. Secure the lid on the specimen container
   c. Use the correct container
   d. All of the above
3. ……………. Is used for routine urinalysis
   a. Midstream specimen
   b. Clean catch specimen
   c. Random urine specimen
   d. Clean voided specimen
4. When collecting …………… the person stops the urine stream, and voids into a sterile specimen
   a. Random urine specimen
   b. Midstream specimen
   c. 24 hour urine specimen
   d. None of the above
5. …………. Prevents growth of microbes in urine
   a. Warming
   b. Chilling
   c. Putting disinfectant
   d. Sterilization
6. A 24-hour urine test is restarted if ………..
   a. A voiding was not saved
   b. Toilet tissue was discarded into the specimen
   c. The specimen contains stools
   d. All of the above
7. Urine can be tested for ………..
   a. Alkaline
   b. Blood
   c. Glucose
   d. All of the above
8. Which of the following is a normal acidic level in urine?
   a. 3.5
   b. 5.0
   c. 10.1
   d. 15.6
9. …………. Means sugar in the urine

a. Ketones

b. Glycerin

c. Glycosuria

d. Glucose

10. Test for glucose and ketones are usually done …….. a day

   a. 2

   b. 3

   c. 4

   d. 5

11. Blood in the urine is known as ……….

   a. Hematuria

   b. Hemasuria

   c. Hemoptysis

   d. Hematone

12. All of the following should be done when using reagent strip EXCEPT

   a. Dip the strip into the urine

   b. Do not touch the test area on the strip

   c. Shake the strip to display color

   d. Compare the strip with the color chart

13. Stools are studied for …………

   a. Fat

   b. Blood

   c. Worms

   d. All of the above

14. Sputum is coughed from the …………..

   a. Bronchi

   b. Lungs

   c. Chest

   d. Heart

15. Which of the following guidelines should be adhered to when collecting sputum specimen?

   a. Perform oral hygiene before collecting sample

   b. Use mouth wash for the patient before collecting specimen

   c. Have the person rinse mouth with water before collecting specimen

   d. All of the above

Section 23

Assisting with exercise and activity

1. Which of the following can limit activity?
    a. Illness
    b. Surgery
    c. Injury
    d. All of the above
2. In ……. everything is done for the person
    a. Strict bedrest
    b. Bedrest
    c. Bedrest with commode privileges
    d. Bedrest with bathroom privileges
3. Which of the following complications can result from bedrest?
    a. Pressure ulcer
    b. Nausea
    c. Vomiting
    d. All of the above
4. A …………..is the lack of joint mobility caused by abnormal shortening of a muscle
    a. Atrophy
    b. Contracture
    c. Orthostatic pressure
    d. Contraction
5. ………… is the decrease in size or the wasting away of tissue
    a. Dorsiflexion
    b. Flexion
    c. Atrophy
    d. Contracture
6. Which of the following is a sign of contracture?
    a. Stiffness
    b. The area is deformed
    c. The skin cannot stretch
    d. All of the above
7. Which of the following is a common site for contracture
    a. Knees
    b. Back
    c. Stomach
    d. All of the above
8. Orthostatic hypotension is abnormally low blood pressure when the person suddenly …………
    a. Shakes legs
    b. Stands up
    c. Lie down
    d. Stretch hands
9. ………….. are placed under the mattress to prevent it from sagging

a. Bed grips

b. Bed cradle

c. Bed boards

d. Bed rolls

10. ....prevents plantar flexion that can lead to foot drop

   a. Foot flexion

   b. Foot boards

   c. Plantar footdrop

   d. Foot rolls

11. Trochanter rolls prevent ....

   a. Contractures of the thumb

   b. Atrophy in the neck

   c. The hips and the legs from turning outwards

   d. All of the above

12. ....keeps the elbow, wrist, thumb, fingers, ankles, and knees in normal position

   a. Splints

   b. Hand grips

   c. Bed cradle

   d. Trochanter rolls

13. In active range of emotions exercise ....

   a. The exercise is done by the person

   b. You help move the joints through their range of motion

   c. The person does the exercise with some help

   d. Exercise is not done

14. .... is moving a body part toward the mid-line of the body

   a. Opposition

   b. Flexion

   c. Adduction

   d. Pronation

15. .... is excessive straightening of a body part

   a. Overextension

   b. Rotation

   c. Supination

   d. Hyperextension

16. Flexion is ....

   a. Bending a body part

   b. Turning the joint

   c. Moving a body part

   d. Straightening the body part

17. Which of the following guidelines should be adhered to when carrying out range of motion exercise with a patient?

   a. Do not force a joint beyond its range of emotion

   b. Ask if he or she feels pain

   c. Do not force a joint to the point of pain

d. All of the above

18. Which of the following activities may be the first to likely occur after bedrest?
    a. Walking
    b. Sitting in the bedside chair
    c. Jogging
    d. Strolling

19. When assisting a patient with ambulation, which of the following should be adhered to?
    a. Ensure that the toe tips strikes the floor first
    b. Walk the required distance even if the patient is tired
    c. Do not rush the person
    d. Stand at the person's strong side to maintain balance

20. Crutches are used in all of the following situation EXCEPT
    a. When a person cannot use one leg
    b. When the both legs are paralyzed
    c. When one leg needs to gain strength
    d. When both legs needs to gain strength

21. Which of the following is a safety measure to be adhered to when using crutches for a patient?
    a. Tighten all bolts
    b. Clothes must be loosed to allow movement of air
    c. Ensure shoes have skid soles
    d. Keep the crutches out of the patients sight

22. Walkers give more support than …………
    a. Wheel chair
    b. Wheeled walkers
    c. Cane
    d. All of the above

23. Which of the following is true about the use of cane?
    a. Canes are used for weakness on one side of the body
    b. They can be used for weakness on the both sides of the body
    c. It is held on the weak side of the body
    d. All of the above

24. Which of the following is a function of braces?
    a. It support weak side of the body
    b. It prevents deformities
    c. It corrects deformities
    d. All of the above

25. Which of the following can be done to promote independence?
    a. Forcing the person to take part in social activities
    b. Activities may not have to meet the person's interest
    c. Encourage resident to share ideas
    d. All of the above

Section 24

Assisting with wound care

1. Which of the following is a common cause of wound?
    a. Surgery
    b. Nerve damage
    c. Trauma
    d. All of the above
2. A wound is ....
    a. Portal of exit for microbes
    b. Portal of entry for microbes
    c. Portal of dwelling for microbes
    d. All of the above
3. Which of the following is a common site for skin tears
    a. Face
    b. Ear
    c. Arms
    d. Stomach
4. Which of the following is a common cause of skin tears?
    a. Removing tapes or adhesives
    b. Stretching too hard
    c. Malnutrition
    d. All of the above
5. Which of the following should be done to prevent skin tears?
    a. Prevent shearing and friction when moving
    b. Keep fingernails short and smoothly filed
    c. Remove tape carefully
    d. All of the above
6. Vascular ulcer is caused by ....
    a. Lack of vitamin C
    b. Decreased blood flow through the veins
    c. Unrelieved pressure
    d. Surgery
7. .... Is a condition in which there is death of tissue
    a. Inflammation
    b. Infection
    c. Gangrene
    d. Ulcer
8. Which of the following is a common site for venous ulcer ?
    a. Forehead
    b. Arm
    c. Heels
    d. Palm
9. Arterial ulcers are found on the ....

a. Lower leg

b. Upper thighs

c. Arm

d. Wrist

10. In diabetes foot ulcer which of the following may occur?

    a. Lose of sensation in the leg

    b. Gangrene

    c. Decreased blood flow

    d. All of the above

11. Which of the following is a function of the elastic stockings

    a. It prevents blood clot

    b. It prevents cracked skin

    c. It prevents hammer toe

    d. All of the above

12. A pulmonary embolism can cause ………….

    a. Thrombus

    b. Embolus

    c. Respiratory problem

    d. Leg blisters

13. Which of the following is at risk for thrombi?

    a. A pregnant person

    b. A person with skin tears

    c. A person with plantar warts

    d. A person experiencing nausea

14. Which of the following can be done to prevent circulatory ulcer?

    a. Encourage crossing of legs while sitting

    b. Do not dress the person tight clothes

    c. Use elastic band type garter to hold stocks in place

    d. Rub the skin while bathing

15. Which of the following should be adhered to when applying bandages?

    a. Start from the proximal part and work towards the dorsal part

    b. Ensure the bandage is very tight

    c. Expose the fingers and toes

    d. All of the above

16. Which of the following is a function of wound dressing?

    a. Absorbs drainage

    b. Prevents bunion

    c. Stops growth of ingrown toenail

    d. Reduces the spread of athlete's foot

17. …………is used for large dressing and frequent dressing changes

    a. Plastic tape

    b. Montgomery ties

    c. Paper tape

    d. Cloth tape

18. Which of the following guidelines should be followed when applying dressing?
    a. Remove the tape pulling it away from the wound
    b. Wet the dressing with dextrose solution
    c. Do not bend or reach over your work area
    d. Change dressing immediately pain relief is administered
19. Which of the following is true about abdominal binders
    a. It provides abdominal support
    b. The top part is at the hips
    c. The lower part is at the thigh
    d. Binders are secured with elastic bands
20. Which of the following is a function of heat on the body?
    a. It relaxes muscles
    b. It relieves pain
    c. It promotes healing
    d. All of the above
21. Which of the following occurs when heat is applied on the skin briefly?
    a. Blood vessels constrict
    b. Blood flow reduces
    c. Tissue have more oxygen and nutrients
    d. Joints become stiff
22. Which of the following complication can occur as a result of applying heat to the skin?
    a. Burns can occur
    b. Inflammation can occur
    c. Infection can occur
    d. Embolus can occur
23. Heat should not be applied on ....
    a. A Pregnant woman's abdomen
    b. Metal implant
    c. Damaged skin
    d. All of the above
24. Which of the following is true about heat application?
    a. Heat penetrates deeper with dry heat application
    b. Water conducts heat
    c. Dry heat has greater and faster effect than moist heat
    d. Dry heat application have lower temperature than moist heat application
25. Burns are more likely with ....
    a. Hot compress
    b. Sitz bath
    c. Dry heat
    d. Hot soak
26. Which of the following is a function of cold application?
    a. Prevents swelling
    b. Relaxes muscles
    c. Dilate blood vessels

    d.   Increase blood flow

27. Prolonged application of cold has which of the following effects?
    a. Blood vessels dilates
    b. Blood flow increases
    c. Tissues have more oxygen
    d. All of the above

28. In a sitz bath, blood flow increase to the …………
    a. Head
    b. Hands
    c. Perineum
    d. Feet

29. Which of the following precautions should be taken when using aquathermia pad?
    a. Place the pad under the person
    b. Prevent the pad from being knocked over
    c. Keep the key used to set the temperature in the patients drawer
    d. All of the above

30. Which of the following ethical rules should be followed?
    a. Taking supplies home for personal use
    b. Charging supplies correctly
    c. Following the agency's rules
    d. All of the above

Section 25

Assisting with pressure ulcers

1. .... is an area where the bone sticks out or projects from the flat surface of the body
   a. Bony prominence
   b. Eschar
   c. Bony structure
   d. Slough prominence
2. ....is when layers of the skin rub against each other
   a. Shear
   b. Friction
   c. Contraction
   d. Pressure
3. Which of the following is also known as pressure ulcers
   a. Decubitus ulcer
   b. Bed sore
   c. Pressure sore
   d. All of the above
4. Which of the following is the major cause of pressure ulcers
   a. Shearing
   b. Friction
   c. Pressure
   d. Fracture
5. Friction does which of the following?
   a. Causes dry skin
   b. Scrapes the skin
   c. Prevent oxygen from reaching cells
   d. Prevents nutrients from reaching the cells
6. Which of the following is at risk for pressure ulcer?
   a. Obese patients
   b. Patients with lowered mental awareness
   c. Patients who have circulatory problems
   d. All of the above
7. At what stage in the pressure ulcer is the skin lost and the subcutaneous fat exposed?
   a. Stage 1
   b. Stage 2
   c. Stage 3
   d. Stage 4
8. Slough may be present in stage ....
   a. 2
   b. 3
   c. 4
   d. 5
9. Which of the following may occur in stage 2?

a. Eschar may be present
b. Slough may be present
c. Subcutaneous fat may be exposed
d. None of the above

10. .... Is thick, leathery dead tissue that may be loose or adhered to the skin
    a. Eschar
    b. Slough
    c. Tendon
    d. Muscle

11. According to center for Medicare and Medicaid services the most common site for pressure ulcer is ....
    a. Breast
    b. Sacrum
    c. Shoulders
    d. Hip

12. Which of the following can be done to prevent pressure ulcers?
    a. Re-position bedfast persons every 5 minutes
    b. Re-position chairfast persons every 5 minutes
    c. Do not position the person on a pressure ulcer
    d. Re-position chairfast person every 4 hours

13. All of the following should be done to the skin to prevent pressure ulcer EXCEPT
    a. Use hot water to bath or clean the skin
    b. Use a cleaning agent as directed
    c. Prevent skin exposure to moisture
    d. Apply moisturizer to dry areas

14. When giving a massage ....
    a. Massage bony areas
    b. Massage when repositioning the person
    c. Massage over pressure points
    d. Massage reddened areas

15. Which of the following clothes should be avoided?
    a. Thick seams and buttons that press against the skin
    b. Tight clothes
    c. Avoid clothes from bunching up
    d. All of the above

16. All of the following should be avoided when giving care to a patient with pressure ulcer EXCEPT
    a. Rubbing the person while drying skin
    b. Applying heat directly on pressure ulcer
    c. Keeping heels and ankles off the bed
    d. Leaving the person on the bedpan longer than needed

17. ....is a metal frame placed on the bed and over the person
    a. Bed cradle
    b. Heel protector
    c. Leg cushions

    d.   Bed cushion
18. ....raises the heel and feet off the bed
    a.   Foot boards
    b.   Trochanter rolls
    c.   Heel and foot elevator
    d.   Bed cradle
19. In special beds the ....
    a.   Person floats on the mattresses
    b.   Person is turned to the prone or supine position
    c.   Pressure points change as the position changes
    d.   All of the above
20. Which of the following occurs if pressure ulcer is colonized?
    a.   There will be delayed healing
    b.   There is risk for osteomyelitis
    c.   Pain is severe
    d.   All of the above

Section 26
Assisting with oxygen needs

1. ....means that the cells do not have enough oxygen
   a. Hypoxia
   b. Cyanosis
   c. Tachypnea
   d. Hyperopia

2. Which of the following is a sign of inadequate oxygen in the brain
   a. Restlessness
   b. Dizziness
   c. Disorientation
   d. All of the above

3. Tachypnea is ....
   a. Slow breathing
   b. Rapid breathing
   c. Lack of breathing
   d. Difficult breathing

4. ....is when breathing is rapid and deeper than normal
   a. Apnea
   b. Hypoxia
   c. Hyperventilation
   d. Orthopnea

5. In .... respirations gradually increases in rate and depth and then becomes shallow and slow
   a. Hypoventilation
   b. Hyperventilation
   c. Cheyne-stokes respiration
   d. Bradypnea

6. Respirations fewer than 12 per minutes is known as ....
   a. Tachypnea
   b. Bradypnea
   c. Orthopenea
   d. Apnea

7. Normal breathe is between .... times per minute
   a. 2 to 5
   b. 5 to 10
   c. 12 to 20
   d. 20 to 25

8. Kussmaul respirations are ....
   a. Very deep and rapid
   b. More than 10 per minute
   c. Difficult and painful
   d. Slow and shallow

9. Air must reach the ....

a. Lungs

b. Alveoli

c. Trachea

d. Bronchi

10. Which of the following interferes with deep breathing?

    a. Pain

    b. Immobility

    c. Drugs

    d. All of the above

11. Breathing is usually easier in …………position

    a. Sims

    b. Fowler's

    c. Supine

    d. Trendelenburg's

12. Position changes are needed at least very …….. hours

    a. 2

    b. 3

    c. 4

    d. 5

13. Which of the following is a benefit of deep breathing and coughing?

    a. It removes mucus

    b. It promotes oxygenation

    c. It strengthens the lungs

    d. All of the above

14. All of the following guidelines should be followed when assisting with deep breathing and coughing exercise EXCEPT?

    a. Encourage the person to cover nose and mouth when coughing

    b. Help the person to a sims position

    c. Have the person inhale through the nose

    d. Ask the person to exhale through the mouth

15. ……… starts and maintains oxygen therapy

    a. Doctor

    b. Nursing assistant

    c. Nurse

    d. Patient

16. Pulse oximetry measures the oxygen concentration in …………blood

    a. Arterial

    b. Vein

    c. Heart

    d. Lungs

17. Oxygen concentration is the percent of ……….. containing oxygen

    a. Vein blood

    b. Hemoglobin

    c. White blood cells

d. Red blood cells

18. The normal range for oxygen concentration is ....
    a. 50% to 60%
    b. 65 % to 70%
    c. 80 to 95%
    d. 95% to 100%

19. Sensor can be attached to .... when measuring oxygen concentration
    a. Finger
    b. Earlobes
    c. Nose
    d. All of the above

20. ....removes oxygen from the air
    a. Oxygen tank
    b. Oxygen concentrator
    c. Liquid oxygen system
    d. Wall outlet

21. The liquid oxygen system has enough oxygen for about ....
    a. 8 hours
    b. 12 hours
    c. 16 hours
    d. 24 hours

22. Which of the following is true about liquid oxygen?
    a. It is warm
    b. It can freeze the skin
    c. It is hot
    d. It should be kept in a warmer

23. Which of the following is true about using oxygen facemask?
    a. It is inserted into the nostrils
    b. Talking and eating is hard
    c. It goes behind the ears and under the chin
    d. All of the above

24. The nursing assistant may ....
    a. Give oxygen
    b. Adjust flow rates
    c. Assist with oxygen therapy
    d. Insert cannula pongs

25. Which of the following safety tips must be adhered to?
    a. Do not remove the oxygen device
    b. Ensure the oxygen device is tight
    c. Puncture tubing to secure it in place
    d. All of the above

Section 27

Assisting with rehabilitation and restorative nursing care

1. ....is any lost or impaired physical or mental function
   a. Disease
   b. Injury
   c. Disability
   d. Birth defect
2. Which of the following is a function of restorative nursing?
   a. Helps maintain the highest level of function
   b. Restores lost mental function
   c. Restores impaired physical function
   d. All of the above
3. Restorative nursing promotes …………
   a. Self-care
   b. Elimination
   c. Positioning
   d. All of the above
4. A …………… is an artificial replacement for a missing body part
   a. Aphasia
   b. Prosthesis
   c. Walker
   d. Crutches
5. Speech therapy is useful in case of …………..
   a. Dyspnea
   b. Apnea
   c. Aphasia
   d. Hypertension
6. All of the following should be done to help patients deal with the psychological effects of disability EXCEPT?
   a. Show pity
   b. Do not argue with the person
   c. Be polite
   d. Listen to the person
7. Which of the following persons is a part of the rehabilitation team?
   a. Family
   b. Nurse
   c. Doctor
   d. All of the above
8. …………rehabilitation program is for patients with heart disorders
   a. Spinal cord
   b. Cardiac
   c. Brain injury
   d. Stroke

9. ....rehabilitation programs is for patients with fractures or joint replacement surgery
   a. Musculo-skeletal
   b. Respiratory
   c. Brain injury
   d. Spinal cord
10. Respiratory rehabilitation is for patients who suffer respiratory disorders like ....
    a. Diabetes
    b. Burns
    c. Lung surgery
    d. Fractures
11. Which of the following must be done to promote quality of life?
    a. Protect the right to privacy
    b. Encourage personal choice
    c. Encourage activities
    d. All of the above
12. Which of the following is allowed when helping a patient rehabilitate?
    a. Screaming at patients
    b. Calling the patient names
    c. Praising the patient for efforts
    d. Striking the patient
13. Restorative aides require which of the following?
    a. Patience
    b. Kindness
    c. Good communication skills
    d. All of the above
14. Which of the following should be stressed in other to promote independence?
    a. The patient's strengths
    b. The patient's weakness
    c. The patient's disabilities
    d. All of the above
15. Which of the following should not be allowed when helping with rehabilitation?
    a. Letting the patient choose activities of interest
    b. Helping the person do things he or she can do
    c. Having the person use self-help device
    d. All of the above

Section 28

Caring for persons with common health problems

1. New growth of abnormal cells is called ....
   a. Cancer
   b. Tumor
   c. Metastasis
   d. Paraplegia
2. ....invade and destroy nearby tissues
   a. Benign tumor
   b. Malignant tumor
   c. Paraplegia tumor
   d. Invasive tumor
3. Which of the following is true about benign tumor?
   a. It is life threatening
   b. It grows back after removal
   c. It does not spread
   d. It is destructive
4. .... is the spread of cancer to other body parts
   a. Tumorsis
   b. Metastasis
   c. Cancer
   d. Hyperplasia
5. Which of the following is a common site for cancer?
   a. Skin
   b. Lungs
   c. Breast
   d. All of the above
6. Cancer is the .... leading cause of death in the united state
   a. First
   b. Second
   c. Third
   d. Fourth
7. Most cancers occur within which of the following age bracket?
   a. 2 to 10 years
   b. 10 to 20 years
   c. 25 to 45 years
   d. 65 years and above
8. Which of the following can cause skin cancer?
   a. Tanning booth
   b. Chewing tobacco
   c. Tobacco smoking
   d. Hormone replacement
9. Which of the following cancer is hereditary?

a. Breast cancer

b. Prostate cancer

c. Ovarian cancer

d. All of the above

10. More than .... Drinks a day of alcohol increases the risk of cancer

   a. 1

   b. 2

   c. 3

   d. 4

11. All of the following cancers can be caused by alcohol EXCCEPT?

   a. Breast cancer

   b. Skin cancer

   c. Liver cancer

   d. Mouth cancer

12. Which of the following increases the risk of cancer?

   a. High fat diet

   b. Lack of physical activities

   c. Being overweight

   d. All of the above

13. Surgery is carried out to .... in cancer treatment

   a. Remove tumor

   b. Disinfect tumor

   c. Kill cells

   d. All of the above

14. Which of the following is a side effect that can occur from the surgery?

   a. Hair loss

   b. Bleeding

   c. Burns

   d. Skin breakdown

15. Which of the following is a sign or symptom of cancer?

   a. Unusual bleeding

   b. Fatigue

   c. Discomfort after eating

   d. All of the above

16. ....is the most common type of arthritis

   a. Osteoarthritis

   b. Rheumatoid arthritis

   c. Osteoporosis

   d. Fracture

17. Which of the following is a cause of degenerative joint disease?

   a. Poor diet

   b. Exposure to Ionizing radiation

   c. Aging

   d. Tobacco smoking

18. Which of the following is true about degenerative joint disease?
    a. It can be cured
    b. It can occur in the thighs
    c. Cold weather increases the symptoms
    d. All of the above

19. A pain relief drug taken for arthritis does which of the following?
    a. Ensure good postures
    b. Decreases swelling
    c. Increases flexibility
    d. None of the above

20. ………….helps with weight control and promotes fitness
    a. Pain relief drugs
    b. Exercise
    c. Cold application
    d. Hot water application

21. ………….is a chronic inflammatory disease
    a. Rheumatoid arthritis
    b. Osteoarthritis
    c. Degenerative joint disease
    d. Osteotomies

22. Which of the following is true about rheumatoid arthritis?
    a. It occurs more in men
    b. It usually develops between the age of 65 to 70
    c. It causes joint pains
    d. All of the above

23. Which of the following is a sign and symptom of rheumatoid arthritis?
    a. Fatigue
    b. Fever
    c. Swollen joints
    d. All of the above

24. All of the following should be done to relieve or reduce rheumatoid arthritis symptoms EXCEPT
    a. Ensure long bed rest
    b. Carry out range of motion exercises
    c. Ensure proper positioning
    d. Provide walking aides

25. Which of the following can help to reduce stress?
    a. Exercise
    b. Relaxation
    c. Wrist and hand splints
    d. All of the above

26. Which of the following care measure should be given after joint replacement surgery?
    a. Ensure deep breathing exercise and coughing
    b. Provide foods and fluids for tissue healing
    c. Provide assistance with walking

d. All of above

27. Which of the following should be avoided after a joint replacement surgery?
    a. Standing straight
    b. Using a high chair with arms
    c. Flexing hips past 90 degrees
    d. Sleeping with pillow between legs

28. With .... the bone becomes porous and brittle
    a. Osteoporosis
    b. Osteotomies
    c. Fracture
    d. Friction

29. Which of the following is true about Osteoporosis?
    a. The bones are broken
    b. Older people are at risk
    c. Americans are more at risk than Asians
    d. All of the above

30. Which of the following is a risk factor for osteoporosis?
    a. Lack of exercise
    b. Falls and accident
    c. Alcohol use
    d. All of the above

31. Which of the following can prevent osteoporosis?
    a. Use of calcium and vitamin supplements
    b. Estrogen supplement for women
    c. Exercise
    d. All of the above

32. In .... the bone is broken but the skin is intact
    a. Open fracture
    b. Compound fracture
    c. Simple fracture
    d. Complex fracture

33. Which of the following guidelines should be followed when providing cast care?
    a. Over the cast with blanket
    b. Turn the person every 2 hours
    c. Place a wet cast on a hard surface
    d. All of the above

34. Casts are made of ....
    a. Plastics
    b. Ropes
    c. Pulleys
    d. Glass

35. Which of the following signs and symptoms should be reported immediately
    a. Pain
    b. Drainage

c. Swelling

d. All of the above

36. When caring for a person in traction ………….

    a. Remove the traction during cleaning

    b. Remove weights after exercise

    c. Check for frayed ropes

    d. Help the person to the toilet for elimination

37. Hip fractures require …………….

    a. Internal fixation

    b. External fixation

    c. Closed reduction

    d. Complex fixation

38. Which of the following should be done when providing care for hip fracture?

    a. Place the chair on the affected side

    b. Allow the person stand on the operated leg if they wish

    c. Apply elastic stockings

    d. All of the above

39. Which of the following can cause loss of limb?

    a. Severe injury

    b. Tumor

    c. Severe infection

    d. All of the above

40. ………… is a condition in which there is death of tissue

    a. Tumors

    b. Gangrene

    c. Vascular disorder

    d. Severe infection

41. Which of the following is true about gangrene?

    a. It can lead to death

    b. Tissues become yellow

    c. Tissues get only oxygen

    d. All of the above

42. Stroke is also called …………..

    a. Brain attack

    b. Hemiplegia

    c. Aphasia

    d. Cerebral blockage

43. Strokes occurs when ………………

    a. A blood vessel is swollen

    b. Bleeding occurs in the brain

    c. Blood clot occurs in the lungs

    d. All of the above

44. Which of the following is a warning sign of stroke?

    a. Sudden weakness of the face

b. Sudden confusion

c. Sudden trouble walking

d. All of the above

45. Which of the following done when caring for a patient with stroke?

    a. Position the person to lie on his face to prevent aspiration

    b. Keep the bed in a semi fowler position

    c. Approach the person from the affected side

    d. All of the above

46. Which of the following is an effect of stroke?

    a. Gangrene

    b. Amputation

    c. Hemiplegia

    d. Hip fracture

47. .... Is difficulty expressing or sending out thoughts

    a. Receptive aphasia

    b. Wernicke's aphasia

    c. Expressive aphasia

    d. Global aphasia

48. Which of the following is true about motor aphasia?

    a. The person knows what to say

    b. He does not understand what is said

    c. The person doesn't know what to say

    d. Objects are not recognized

49. In .... the person has difficulty understanding language

    a. Expressive aphasia

    b. Receptive aphasia

    c. Broca's aphasia

    d. Motor aphasia

50. Which of the following is true about Wernicke's aphasia?

    a. The person understands what is said

    b. People are recognized

    c. The person may not know how to use fork

    d. Thinking is clear

51. In .... the person has problems speaking and understanding language

    a. Mixed aphasia

    b. Joint aphasia

    c. Correlated aphasia

    d. Receptive aphasia

52. Which of the following is true about Parkinson's disease?

    a. It has no cure

    b. Movement is affected

    c. Persons over the age of 50 are at risk

    d. All of the above

53. Which of the following is true about multiple sclerosis?

a. It is not a chronic disease

b. It can be cured

c. Nerve impulses are not sent to and fro the brain normally

d. Symptoms usually start at age 10

54. Which of the following is a sign and symptom of multiple sclerosis?

a. Blurred vision

b. Muscle weakness

c. Pain

d. All of the above

55. ………………is a disease that attacks the nerve cells that control voluntary muscles?

a. Multiple sclerosis

b. Amyotrophic lateral sclerosis

c. Brain damage

d. Paralysis

56. Which of the following is true about Lou Gehrig's disease?

a. Some people affected live for 10 years and more

b. It is more common in women

c. It usually strikes from age 65 and above

d. Most die 1 or 2 years after onset

57. Lou Gehrig's disease affects ………….

a. Motor nerve cells in the brain

b. Bowel function

c. Hearing function

d. Intelligence

58. Traumatic brain injury occurs when …………

a. The muscles in the scalp weakens

b. Cells stop sending messages to the muscles

c. A sudden trauma damages the brain

d. Brain cannot voluntary start movement

59. Which of the following is true for head injury?

a. Brain tissue is bruised or torn

b. Bleeding can occur in the brain

c. Spinal cord injuries are likely

d. All of the above

60. Which of the following can occur as a result of head injury?

a. Cognitive problems

b. Sensory problems

c. Communication problem

d. All of the above

61. …………… is when the person is unconscious and unaware of surroundings. He or she has a sleep wake cycle and periods of being alert.

a. Stupor

b. Coma

c. Vegetative state

d. Persistent vegetative state

62. A person is said to be in .... If he is unresponsive, but can be briefly aroused
    a. Coma
    b. Stupor
    c. Vegetative state
    d. Persistent vegetative state

63. .... Is paralysis in the legs and lower trunk
    a. Paraplegia
    b. Quadriplegia
    c. Tetraplegia
    d. None of the above

64. Which of the following is a common cause of paralysis?
    a. Gunshot wounds
    b. Tobacco use
    c. Exposure to radiation
    d. Excessive alcohol intake

65. Which of the following a sign and symptom of hear loss?
    a. Leaning forward to hear
    b. Speaking too loudly
    c. Asking for words to be repeated
    d. All of the above

66. Hearing aides are used to ....
    a. Restore hearing
    b. Cure hearing problems
    c. Make background noise and speech louder
    d. Correct hearing problems

67. Which of the following can be done to promote hearing?
    a. Approach the person from behind
    b. Shout when talking
    c. Reduce background noise
    d. Keep lengthy conversations

68. ....is a clouding of the lens
    a. Macular mucus
    b. Cataract
    c. Retinopathy
    d. Glaucoma

69. Which of the following is true about age related macular degeneration?
    a. It causes blind spot in the center of vision
    b. It cannot be cured
    c. It is common in men than women
    d. All of the above

70. ....results when fluid builds up in the eye and causes pressure on the optic nerve
    a. Cataract
    b. Glaucoma

c. Age related macular degeneration

d. Diabetic retinopathy

71. Which of the following is true about glaucoma?

a. Prior damage can be reversed

b. Drugs can control glaucoma

c. Peripheral vision is not lost

d. All of the above

72. All of the following nursing measures should be carried out after cataract surgery EXCEPT

a. Keep the eye shield in place as directed

b. Do not bump the eye

c. Place the over-bed table and bedside stand on the operative side

d. Ensure the shield is worn to sleep

73. Which of the following is true about Braille?

a. The last 10 letters also represents the numbers 0 through 9

b. It is read by moving hands from the right to the left along the line of Braille

c. Braille is read by moving the hands from the left to right along the line of Braille

d. All of the above

74. Which of the following should be done when caring for blind and visually impaired persons?

a. Report worn carpeting and other flooring

b. Do not re-arrange furniture and equipment

c. Keep drawers fully closed

d. All of the above

75. When caring for a person that is blind and visually impaired ....

a. Have the person wear comfortable shoes

b. Provide visual and adaptive device

c. Walk at a normal pace

d. All of the above

76. ....is when the systolic pressure is between 120 and 139 mm Hg

a. Hypertension

b. Pre-hypertension

c. Hypotension

d. Pre-hypotension

77. Which of the following is true about hypertension?

a. It can lead to stroke

b. It can be cured

c. Smoking is allowed but alcohol is not

d. All of the above

78. ....is the most common cause of coronary heart disease

a. Atherosclerosis

b. Angina

c. Gland tumors

d. Head injuries

79. ....is a major complication of coronary heart disease

a. Irregular heart beats

b. Hypertension

c. Hypotension

d. All of the above

80. All of the following is true about cardiovascular disorders EXCEPT

    a. Being overweight is a risk factor

    b. Atherosclerosis can be stopped

    c. Women are at a greater risk than men

    d. Excessive alcohol is a risk factor

81. ....is chest pain from reduced blood flow to part of the heart muscles

    a. Atherosclerosis

    b. Angina

    c. Myocardial infarction

    d. Heart attack

82. Which of the following increases the hearts need for more oxygen?

    a. Exertion

    b. A heavy meal

    c. Stress

    d. All of the above

83. Which of the following is true about myocardial infarction?

    a. Part of the lung muscles dies

    b. Blood pumping from the lungs is reduced

    c. Sudden cardiac death can occur

    d. The resting blood pressure is high

84. Myocardial infarction is also called ....

    a. Acute coronary infarction

    b. Acute myocardial syndrome

    c. Heart attack

    d. Angina

85. Which of the following is a sign and symptom of myocardial infarction?

    a. Chest pain

    b. Dyspnea

    c. Nausea

    d. All of the above

86. ....occurs when the weakened heart cannot pump normally

    a. Pulmonary edema

    b. Congestive heart failure

    c. Liver congestion

    d. Heart attack

87. Which of the following is true about heart failure?

    a. The body does not get enough blood

    b. Blood pressure increases

    c. More blood is pumped to the lungs

    d. All of the above

88. Which of the following is a sign and symptom of heart failure?

a. Dyspnea

b. Increased sputum

c. Cough

d. All of the above

89. Which of the following can be done in case of a heart failure?

a. A sodium controlled diet is ordered

b. Sims position is preferred

c. Drugs are administered to increase fluid in the body

d. All of the above

90. Chronic obstructive pulmonary disease involves .... disorders

a. 2

b. 3

c. 4

d. 5

91. ....is the best way to prevent Chronic obstructive pulmonary disease

a. Exercising

b. Eating balanced diet

c. Not smoking

d. Not drinking alcohol

92. ....is often the first symptoms of chronic bronchitis

a. Nausea

b. Vomiting

c. Dyspnea

d. Smoker's cough

93. Which of the following is true about chronic bronchitis?

a. Smoking is a major cause

b. The body does not get normal amounts of oxygen

c. The person may cough up mucus

d. All of the above

94. In .... The alveoli enlarge

a. Asthma

b. Emphysema

c. Influenza

d. Chronic bronchitis

95. .... Is the most common cause of emphysema?

a. Allergies

b. Cold air

c. Smoking

d. Exertion

96. Which of the following is true about emphysema?

a. The alveoli become more elastic

b. Some air is trapped inside the alveoli during exhaling

c. Trapped air are exhaled in few seconds

d. The person easily breathes in but not out

97. Asthma is usually triggered by ....
   a. Allergies
   b. Coughing
   c. Smoking
   d. Infections

98. Influenza is a respiratory infection caused by ....
   a. Bacteria
   b. Viruses
   c. Infection
   d. Allergies

99. Which of the following is a sign of flu?
   a. High fever
   b. Headache
   c. Chest discomfort
   d. All of the above

100.   .... is an inflammation and infection of lung tissue
   a. Influenza
   b. Asthma
   c. Pneumonia
   d. Tuberculosis

101.   Which of the following is a cause of pneumonia?
   a. Bacteria
   b. Viruses
   c. Microbes
   d. All of the above

102.   ....is a symptom and sign of pneumonia
   a. High fever
   b. Muscle aches
   c. Chills
   d. All of the above

103.   Which of the following should be done in case of pneumonia?
   a. Decrease fluid intake
   b. Ensure the patient does mild exercises
   c. Oxygen may be needed
   d. All of the above

104.   Which of the following is true about tuberculosis?
   a. It is spread by airborne droplets with cough
   b. People nearby can inhale the virus
   c. It is a viral infection
   d. Infection occurs in the trachea

105.   Which of the following is a sign and symptom of TB?
   a. Weight loss
   b. Vomiting
   c. Depression

d. Anxiety

106. A TB patient should take which of the following precautions?
a. The person must cover mouth and nose with tissue when sneezing
b. Hand washing should be carried out
c. Tissues should be flushed down the toilet
d. All of the above

107. Which of the following is true about vomiting?
a. It signals illness
b. It is caused by small pouches in the colon
c. It is caused by stomach inflammation
d. Airway should be blocked to reduce vomit

108. Recovery of hepatitis takes about............
a. 2 days
b. 1 week
c. 2 weeks
d. 1 month

109. .... is spread by the fecal oral route
a. Hepatitis B
b. Hepatitis C
c. Hepatitis A
d. Hepatitis D

110. Hepatitis B is spread through ....
a. Kissing
b. Anal sex
c. Breast feeding
d. Coughing

111. Which of the following is a cause of hepatitis A?
a. Poor nutrition
b. Poor sanitation
c. Crowded living condition
d. All of the above

112. Which of the following is true about hepatitis C?
a. Liver disease may show up later
b. A person without symptoms cannot transmit the disease
c. It can be transmitted by persons with hepatitis B
d. All of the above

113. Hepatitis D occurs only in people infected with hepatitis ....
a. A
b. B
c. C
d. D

114. Which of the following is not common in the United States?
a. Hepatitis B
b. Hepatitis C

c. Hepatitis E

d. Hepatitis D

115. Which of the following is a sign or symptom of hepatitis?

a. Jaundice

b. Fatigue

c. Diarrhea

d. All of the above

116. Which of the following is a common cause of urinary tract infection

a. Poor perineal hygiene

b. Immobility

c. Intercourse

d. All of the above

117. .... is a bladder infection caused by bacteria

a. Pyelonephritis

b. Cystitis

c. Calculi

d. Kidney failure

118. Which of the following is true about pyelonephritis?

a. It can lead to cystitis

b. Urine may contain pus

c. It is caused by bacteria

d. It is a viral infection

119. Which of the following is a sign and symptom of cystitis?

a. Foul smelling urine

b. Sneezing

c. Thick sputum

d. Painful cough

120. A patient with kidney stone has to drink .... of water a day

a. 500ml to 1000ml

b. 1000ml to 2000ml

c. 2000ml to 3000ml

d. 4000ml to 6000ml

121. Which of the following is a risk factor for calculi?

a. Bedrest

b. Poor fluid intake

c. Immobility

d. All of the above

122. .... is a sign or symptom of kidney stones

a. Dysuria

b. Dyspnea

c. Cyanosis

d. Muscle ache

123. The prostate lies in front of the ....

a. Colon

b. Rectum

c. Bladder

d. Penis

124. Which of the following is true about benign prostatic hyperplasia?

a. It occurs usually in men after the age of 60

b. It obstruct urine flow

c. Bladder function is gradually lost

d. All of the above

125. Sexually transmitted diseases is spread through …………

a. Oral sex

b. Vaginal sex

c. Anal sex

d. All of the above

126. Sexually transmitted disease can occur in the …………

a. Genital areas

b. Ears

c. Nose

d. All of the above

127. ………….. is the most common endocrine disorder

a. Adrenal cancer

b. Hypoglycemia

c. Diabetes

d. Addison's disease

128. Which of the following is true about diabetes?

a. Cells have too much sugar

b. Sugar builds up in the blood

c. The body can produce insulin and can also use it properly

d. All of the above

129. …………. Occurs most often in children

a. Type 1 diabetes

b. Type 2 diabetes

c. Gestational diabetes

d. Type 3 diabetes

130. In type 1 diabetes …..

a. Onset is slow

b. The pancreas produce little or no insulin

c. The pancreas secretes insulin

d. Healing takes place within 1 month

131. Which of the following is true about type 2 diabetes?

a. It is more common in young adults

b. Onset is rapid

c. The body cannot use insulin well

d. All of the above

132. Which of the following is a sign and symptom of diabetes?

a. Urinating often
b. Pus in the urine
c. Yellow sputum
d. All of the above

133. ....is a complication that may occur from diabetes
a. Stroke
b. Heart attack
c. Blindness
d. All of the above

134. Which of the following should be done to control diabetes?
a. Over-weight person need to lose weight
b. Good foot care is needed
c. Blood glucose should be monitored daily
d. All of the above

135. Which of the following is a common autoimmune system disorder?
a. Lupus
b. Hypoglycemia
c. Acquired immunodeficiency syndrome
d. Hypertrophy

136. .... is when the thyroid glands produce too much thyroid hormone
a. Reactive arthritis
b. Hashimoto's thyroiditis
c. Graves' disease
d. Chronic thyroiditis

137. .... is an inflammatory disease affecting the blood cells, joints, skin, kidney, lungs, heart, or brain
a. Acquired immunodeficiency syndrome
b. Lupus
c. Heart failure
d. Stroke

138. Human immunodeficiency virus is spread through ....
a. Sneezing
b. Breast milk
c. Saliva
d. All of the above

139. Persons with AIDS are at risk for ....
a. Pneumonia
b. Nervous system damage
c. Paralysis
d. All of the above

140. Which of the following is a sign of AIDS?
a. Depression
b. Fatigue
c. Weight loss

d. All of the above

Section 29

Caring for persons with mental health disorders

1. ....is a vague uneasy feeling in response to stress
   a. Phobia
   b. Anxiety
   c. Panic
   d. Denial

2. Which of the following is a healthy way of dealing with anxiety?
   a. Eating
   b. Exercising
   c. Playing music
   d. Taking a hot bath

3. In .... the person worries about health, money, or family problems
   a. Panic anxiety
   b. Generalized anxiety
   c. Post-traumatic stress disorder
   d. None of the above

4. ....is an intense and sudden feeling of fear, anxiety, terror or dread
   a. Anxiety
   b. Phobia
   c. Panic disorder
   d. Fear

5. Which of the following is a symptom of anxiety?
   a. Loss of appetite
   b. Diarrhea
   c. Sweating
   d. All of the above

6. Phobia means intense ....
   a. Fear
   b. Anxiety
   c. Depression
   d. Pulse

7. Fear of uncleanliness is ....
   a. Agoraphobia
   b. Mysophobia
   c. Claustrophobia
   d. Aquaphobia

8. ....is a recurrent, unwanted thought, idea or image
   a. Obsession
   b. Repetition
   c. Compulsion
   d. Anxiety

9. ....occurs after a terrifying event

a. Compulsion

b. Phobia

c. Post-traumatic stress disorder

d. Anxiety

10. Which of the following is a defense mechanism?

a. Repressing the thoughts of being sexually assaulted

b. Acting in a way that is opposite to what you feel

c. Yelling at your friend while angry at your boss

d. All of the above

11. Which of the following is a sign and symptom of post-traumatic stress disorder?

a. Aggressive and violent behaviors

b. Irritability

c. Flashbacks

d. All of the above

12. .... is seeing, hearing, smelling, or feeling something that is not real

a. Paranoia

b. Hallucination

c. Delusions

d. Thought disorders

13. A person is suffering from ....if he believes that the newspaper is talking about him or referring to him

a. Bipolar disorder

b. Paranoia

c. Delusions

d. Hallucination

14. Delusion of persecution are false beliefs of being ....

a. A super hero

b. Mistreated

c. Important

d. A celebrity

15. A person always suspicious of others has ....

a. Paranoia

b. Emotional problems

c. Cognitive problems

d. Bipolar disorder

16. Which of the following is true about thought disorders?

a. The person has trouble organizing thought

b. Speech may be garbled

c. The person may suddenly stop speaking in the middle of a thought

d. All of the above

17. A person with .... may have problem understanding or remembering information

a. Movement disorder

b. Cognitive problems

c. Emotional problems

d. Behavioral problems
18. Which of the following is true about schizophrenia?
    a. The onset tends to be earlier in women than men
    b. Symptoms usually begin between the ages of 16 to 30
    c. People with schizophrenia are violent
    d. All of the above
19. Which of the following guidelines should be observed when attending to a patient with schizophrenia?
    a. Try to convince the person that the situation is not real
    b. Tell the person you can see or hear the same thing
    c. Speak slowly and calmly
    d. All of the above
20. A person with …………. has severe extremes in mood, energy and ability to function
    a. Bipolar disorder
    b. Depression
    c. Emotional problems
    d. Paranoia
21. Which of the following is true about depression?
    a. It involves the body only
    b. Physical disorders can cause depression
    c. It does not run in the family
    d. All of the above
22. Which of the following is a sign and symptom of a manic episodes?
    a. Sadness
    b. Poor judgement
    c. Guilt
    d. All of the above
23. ……….is a sign and symptom of depressive episodes?
    a. Suicide attempt
    b. Aggressive behavior
    c. Increased sex drive
    d. Spending sprees
24. Which of the following is a cause of depression?
    a. Loss of job
    b. Death of partner
    c. Loss of body function
    d. All of the above
25. Which of the following shows antisocial personality disorder?
    a. The person lacks responsibility and has no guilt
    b. The person has sleeping problems
    c. The person feels like a super hero
    d. All of the above
26. …….. involves unstable moods, behaviors, and relationships
    a. Bipolar disorder

b. Borderline personality disorder

c. Paranoia

d. Antisocial personality disorder

27. Which of the following is true about alcoholism?

a. It can damage the brain overtime

b. It is a terminal disease

c. It can be cured

d. All of the above

28. Which of the following is true about drug abuse and addiction?

a. Higher doses are usually needed

b. Prolonged use can lead to stroke

c. Treatment is a long process

d. All of the above

29. A person with anorexia nervosa ………..

a. Eats large amount of food

b. Eats out of control

c. Avoids food

d. Loves eating fast food

30. which of the following is a risk factor for suicide?

a. Depression

b. Family history of suicide

c. Incarceration

d. All of the above

Section 30

Caring for persons with confusion and dementia

1. ……………is a mental state of being disoriented to person, time, place, situation, or identity
   a. Dementia
   b. Confusion
   c. Depression
   d. Apprehension
2. Which of the following is a cause of confusion?
   a. Brain injury
   b. Disease
   c. Infections
   d. All of the above
3. Which of the following is true about confusion?
   a. Confusion from physical changes can still be cured
   b. Memory and ability to make good judgments are lost
   c. With aging blood supply to the brain will increase
   d. Acute confusion occurs slowly
4. ………..is the loss of cognitive function that interferes with routine personal, social and occupational activities
   a. Depression
   b. Confusion
   c. Dementia
   d. Delirium
5. Early warning signs of dementia include ……….
   a. Memory loss
   b. Drugs and alcohol
   c. Tumors
   d. All of the above
6. ……………is the most common type of permanent dementia
   a. Alzheimer's
   b. Pseudo dementia
   c. Delirium
   d. Depression
7. Which of the following is true about delirium?
   a. It is permanent
   b. It cannot be reversed
   c. It often lasts for about one week
   d. All of the above
8. Which of the following is a cause of permanent dementia?
   a. Brain tumors
   b. Stroke
   c. Syphilis
   d. All of the above

9. ....is the most common mental health disorder in older persons
   a. Dementia
   b. Delirium
   c. Depression
   d. Alzheimer's disease
10. Which of the following is true about Alzheimer's disease?
   a. It is a brain disease
   b. There is a steady decline in memory
   c. Onset is gradual
   d. All of the above
11. First symptoms of Alzheimer's disease first appear after age ....
   a. 60
   b. 40
   c. 30
   d. 25
12. Which of the following is false about Alzheimer's disease?
   a. It is a normal part of aging
   b. More women than men have it
   c. Nearly half of persons age 85 and older have Alzheimer's disease
   d. The cause is unknown
13. Which of the following is the classic sign of Alzheimer's disease?
   a. Gradual loss of short term memory
   b. Neglects to bath
   c. Misplacing household items
   d. Taking longer to do things
14. In mild Alzheimer's disease which of the following occurs?
   a. Cannot communicate
   b. Seizures
   c. Poor judgement
   d. Hallucination
15. Which of the following occurs in moderate Alzheimer's disease?
   a. Getting lost
   b. Delusions
   c. Repeating questions
   d. Problems handling money
16. Which of the following precautions should be taken when taking care of patients who wander?
   a. Alert other staff members
   b. Allow the patient to wander in safe enclosed gardens
   c. Guide the person who wanders to a safe area
   d. All of the above
17. Which of the following is true about sundowning?
   a. Symptoms of Alzheimer disease increases when there is sunshine
   b. Symptoms increases when the patients are sitting in the garden
   c. Behavior is worse when the sun goes down

    d.   The person is afraid of sunlight

18. …………are extreme responses to normal events or things
    a. Agitation
    b. Aggression
    c. Catastrophic reactions
    d. Hallucinations

19. A person with AD may ……….
    a. Forget what he or she wants to say
    b. Say the same thing over and over
    c. Hide things
    d. All of the above

20. Which of the following should be done when communicating with a patient with AD?
    a. Use a baby voice
    b. Avoid frowning
    c. Correct the patient carefully
    d.   All of the above

Section 31

Assisting with emergency care

1. Which of the followings rules should be adhered to when giving emergency care?
   a. Stay calm
   b. Lift the person up from where you found him
   c. Give the person fluids
   d. All of the above
2. The goals of first aid is to ....
   a. Prevent death
   b. Call fire department
   c. Move the person to the hospital
   d. Keep the person warm
3. Which of the following can be done to activate Emergency Medical Service?
   a. Dial 911
   b. Call the local fire department
   c. Call the phone operator
   d. All of the above
4. A person is clinically dead.........
   a. When respiration is slow
   b. When heart beat is rapid
   c. When the heart stops
   d. When blood circulation is low
5. Which of the following is a chain of survival for adults?
   a. Activating EMS at once
   b. Early defibrillation
   c. Early cardiopulmonary resuscitation
   d. All of the above
6. .... is when the heart stops suddenly and without warning
   a. Respiratory arrest
   b. Cardiac arrest
   c. Clinical death
   d. Chest compression
7. Which of the following is a major sign of sudden cardiac arrest?
   a. There is no response from the person
   b. The skin is pale
   c. The person is not moving
   d. All of the above
8. Which of the following is true about cardiac arrest?
   a. Agonal respiration may occur
   b. It is an expected event
   c. The heart pumps blood in excess amount
   d. All of the above

9. Which of the following is true about respiratory arrest?
   a. Breathing is rapid and heavy
   b. The heart stops for several minutes
   c. It can lead to cardiac arrest
   d. None of the above
10. Rescue breaths are given ………….
    a. When the person is clinically dead
    b. When there is a pulse but no breathing
    c. When the heart stops
    d. There is no pulse and no heart beat
11. Which of the following is true about cardiopulmonary resuscitation?
    a. It supports circulation and breathing
    b. It provides blood and oxygen to the heart
    c. It must be started at once
    d. All of the above
12. Chest compressions does which of the following?
    a. Forces blood through the circulatory system
    b. Allows air to flow into the body
    c. Transfers air to the brain
    d. Forces air into the lungs
13. Which of the following procedures should be followed when performing chest compressions?
    a. Ensure the person is fully clothed for privacy
    b. Use the heel of your hands when performing the procedure
    c. For effectiveness place the person in a semi-fowler position
    d. All of the above
14. Which of the following is a recommendation from the American Heart Association?
    a. Push hard and fast
    b. Push deeply into the chest
    c. Give compression at a rate of at least 100 per minute
    d. All of the above
15. Which of the following is a benefit of using barrier device for giving breaths?
    a. It is faster than mouth to mouth
    b. It is allows air to move in deeper
    c. It reduces the risk of infection
    d. All of the above
16. Which of the following stops ventricular fibrillation?
    a. Mouth to mouth breathing
    b. Defibrillator
    c. Barrier device breathing
    d. Chest compression
17. Which of the following is true about ventricular fibrillation?
    a. It causes sudden cardiac arrest
    b. The heart produces abnormal rhythm
    c. The heart does not pump blood

d. All of the above

18. Cardiopulmonary resuscitation is done for …………
    a. Fainting
    b. Collapsing
    c. Cardiac arrest
    d. All of the above

19. Which of the following is a sign of cardiac arrest?
    a. The person has a pulse
    b. The person lies still breathing normally
    c. There is no breathing
    d. There is breathing but heart is not pumping blood

20. A recovery position is used when …………..
    a. There is a pulse
    b. The person is not breathing
    c. The person has neck injuries
    d. The person is not responding

21. Which of the following is true about choking?
    a. It can lead to cardiac arrest
    b. Air cannot pass through the lungs
    c. The body does not get enough oxygen
    d. All of the above

22. Which of the following can be used to relieve severe airway obstruction
    a. Defibrillator
    b. Abdominal thrust
    c. Mouth to mouth breathing
    d. Chest compressions

23. All of the following is true about hemorrhage EXCEPT?
    a. It occurs only externally
    b. It can cause death
    c. The larger the blood vessels the greater the bleeding
    d. It cannot be cured

24. Which of the following should be done in case of hemorrhage?
    a. Administer fluids
    b. Remove the object that stabbed the person
    c. Place a clean material over the wound
    d. Remove the dressing if soaked with blood

25. Which of the following can cause fainting?
    a. Hunger
    b. Fatigue
    c. Fear
    d. All of the above

26. Which of the following can cause shock?
    a. Loss of blood
    b. Heart attack

c. Burns

d. All of the above

27. ....is a life threatening sensitivity to an antigen

a. Fainting

b. Shock

c. Anaphylaxis

d. Seizures

28. Which of the following is true about anaphylactic shock?

a. Reactions can occur within seconds

b. It is not an emergency

c. It can be caused by burns

d. All of the above

29. ....occurs when the brain is suddenly deprived of its blood supply

a. Shock

b. Stroke

c. Seizures

d. Anaphylactic shock

30. Which of the following is true about stroke?

a. It usually affects the whole brain

b. There can be loss of consciousness

c. An itchy rash usually occurs

d. All of the above

31. In .... only one part of the brain is involved

a. Generalized tonic-clonic seizure

b. Partial seizures

c. Generalized absence seizures

d. Generalized seizures

32. In the tonic phase ....

a. The person loses consciousness

b. Muscles groups and relax

c. Jerking occurs

d. All of the above

33. ....usually lasts a few seconds

a. Partial seizures

b. Generalized tonic-clonic seizures

c. Generalized absence seizures

d. Generalized seizures

34. Which of the following is true about seizures?

a. Movements are uncontrolled

b. The persons may lose consciousness

c. Lack of blood flow to the brain can cause seizures

d. All of the above

35. Which of the following is an emergency care for seizures?

a. Try to stop the seizure

b. Put an object between the person's teeth
c. Do not leave the person alone
d. All of the above

Section 32

Assisting with end of life care

1. An illness from which the person is not likely to recover is a ....
   a. Terminal illness
   b. Critical illness
   c. Acute illness
   d. Chronic illness
2. Which of the following is the intent of a palliative care?
   a. To provide cure
   b. To reduce the intensity of the symptoms
   c. To treat the illness
   d. All of the above
3. Persons in hospice care usually have less than .... to live
   a. 1 week
   b. 6 months
   c. 2 years
   d. 5 years
4. Which of the following is true about hospice care?
   a. Cure is not provided
   b. Pain relief is stressed
   c. The goal is to improve quality of life
   d. All of the above
5. Attitudes about death is based on ....
   a. Culture
   b. Age
   c. Religion
   d. All of the above
6. According to Dr. Elisabeth's stages of grief, stage 1 is ......
   a. Denial
   b. Anger
   c. Depression
   d. Hopelessness
7. In stage 2 the person thinks ....
   a. No, not me
   b. Why me
   c. Yes it happening to me
   d. This is a mistake
8. In the bargaining stage, the person ....
   a. Is angry
   b. Bargains with God
   c. Envy those with life and health
   d. Is at peace

9. In the acceptance stage, the person ....
    a. Completes unfinished businesses
    b. Accepts death
    c. Is at peace
    d. All of the above
10. All of the following are ways of communicating with patients who are dying EXCEPT
    a. Listening to them
    b. Telling them you know how it feels
    c. Touching them to show care
    d. Be with them
11. Which of the following is a common end of life problem?
    a. Dyspnea
    b. Noisy breathing
    c. Pain
    d. All of the above
12. Which of the following should be done when giving care to dying patients?
    a. Talk about the person when you are giving care
    b. Allow bright light in the room
    c. Speak to the person
    d. If the person cannot talk, do not speak to them
13. When giving end of life care ....
    a. Force the patient to eat at least 3 times a day
    b. Ensure the room is dark when they are sleeping
    c. Remove unnecessary equipment from the room
    d. Even if there is no sign of cold, provide blankets to keep the patient warm
14. Do not resuscitate orders means ....
    a. The person is allowed to die with peace and dignity
    b. The person cannot make his or her own decisions
    c. The person appoints a health proxy
    d. The person should be revived with CPR
15. Which of the following is a sign of death?
    a. Heavy perspiration
    b. Circulation fails
    c. Sensation is lost
    d. All of the above

Section 1

Hospitals and nursing centers

1. B
2. C
3. B
4. A
5. D
6. A
7. C
8. D
9. D
10. B
11. A
12. A
13. C
14. D
15. B
16. C
17. C
18. A
19. D
20. B
21. B
22. A
23. C
24. B
25. B
26. A
27. B
28. D
29. C
30. D

Section 2
The person's right
1. B
2. A
3. D
4. D
5. C
6. B
7. A

8. A
9. B
10. D
11. B
12. C
13. D
14. A
15. C

Section 3

The nursing assistant

1. D
2. D
3. A
4. C
5. B
6. D
7. A
8. C
9. B
10. D
11. A
12. C
13. D
14. A
15. C
16. B
17. C
18. A
19. D
20. D
21. B
22. C
23. B
24. A
25. C
26. A
27. D
28. B

29. D
30. A

Section 4

Work ethics

1. A
2. B
3. A
4. C
5. D
6. B
7. C
8. D
9. B
10. D
11. B
12. A
13. A
14. C
15. D
16. A
17. D
18. B
19. D
20. D
21. A
22. C
23. B
24. D
25. A

Section 5

Communicating with the health team

1. A
2. C
3. D
4. C
5. A
6. D
7. B

8. C
9. D
10. B
11. D
12. A
13. C
14. B
15. D
16. A
17. B
18. C
19. A
20. D
21. C
22. A
23. C
24. B
25. A
26. B
27. D
28. C
29. D
30. A

Section 6

Understanding the person

1. A
2. B
3. D
4. C
5. B
6. A
7. B
8. D
9. A
10. D
11. B
12. C
13. A
14. D
15. B
16. C

17. D
18. C
19. A
20. D

Section 7

Body function and structure

1. A
2. B
3. C
4. A
5. D
6. A
7. C
8. B
9. B
10. A
11. C
12. A
13. B
14. C
15. B
16. A
17. C
18. A
19. B
20. B
21. D
22. C
23. B
24. A
25. C
26. B
27. B
28. A
29. C
30. A
31. D
32. D
33. B
34. A

35. B
36. D
37. B
38. A
39. D
40. C
41. A
42. C
43. B
44. C
45. C
46. A
47. B
48. C
49. A
50. C
51. B
52. A
53. D
54. A
55. C
56. A
57. B
58. A
59. C
60. B
61. D
62. A
63. C
64. B
65. C
66. A
67. D
68. A
69. B
70. C
71. A
72. B
73. B
74. C
75. B
76. C
77. D
78. B

79. D
80. C
81. A
82. B
83. B
84. D
85. A
86. C
87. B
88. C
89. A
90. B
91. D
92. A
93. D
94. B
95. C
96. A
97. A
98. D
99. B
100.   C
101.   A
102.   B
103.   D
104.   B
105.   A
106.   C
107.   D
108.   B
109.   B
110.   C
111.   A
112.   C
113.   D
114.   A
115.   A
116.   D
117.   D
118.   B
119.   C
120.   C
121.   A
122.   B

123.	C
124.	B
125.	D
126.	D
127.	A
128.	C
129.	B
130.	D
131.	C
132.	A
133.	C
134.	C
135.	B

Section 8

Care of the older person

1. A
2. D
3. C
4. A
5. D
6. C
7. C
8. C
9. A
10. A
11. B
12. D
13. A
14. D
15. D

Section 9

Assisting with safety

1. D
2. A
3. B
4. D
5. C

6. D
7. C
8. D
9. A
10. C
11. B
12. D
13. B
14. C
15. A
16. D
17. B
18. C
19. A
20. D
21. C
22. D
23. A
24. A
25. D

Section 10

Assisting with fall prevention

1. D
2. B
3. D
4. C
5. A
6. D
7. A
8. C
9. A
10. B
11. C
12. A
13. D
14. B
15. B

Section 11

Restraint alternatives and safe restraint use

1. A
2. C
3. D
4. B
5. C
6. D
7. A
8. B
9. D
10. C
11. D
12. B
13. C
14. A
15. A
16. C
17. B
18. C
19. A
20. B
21. A
22. C
23. D
24. C
25. D

Section 12

Preventing infection

1. B
2. D
3. C
4. A
5. A
6. B
7. C
8. B
9. B
10. A
11. C

12. D
13. B
14. D
15. A
16. D
17. C
18. D
19. D
20. B
21. C
22. B
23. B
24. A
25. C
26. B
27. D
28. B
29. D
30. A
31. C
32. C
33. B
34. D
35. B
36. A
37. C
38. B
39. A
40. D
41. A
42. B
43. C
44. A
45. D

Section 13

Body mechanics

1. D
2. A
3. B
4. A
5. D

6. B
7. C
8. B
9. A
10. D
11. C
12. B
13. C
14. C
15. B

Section 14

Assisting with moving and transfers

1. B
2. C
3. A
4. B
5. A
6. C
7. D
8. A
9. D
10. C
11. A
12. D
13. A
14. D
15. C
16. B
17. C
18. A
19. D
20. D
21. B
22. C
23. B
24. D
25. D

Section 15

Assisting with comfort

1. D
2. C
3. D
4. B
5. A
6. C
7. A
8. B
9. D
10. A
11. B
12. C
13. C
14. A
15. A
16. B
17. B
18. C
19. D
20. D
21. A
22. D
23. B
24. D
25. C

Section 16

Assisting with hygiene

1. B
2. D
3. A
4. C
5. B
6. D
7. D
8. C

9. A
10. B
11. A
12. C
13. B
14. D
15. B

Section 17

Assisting with grooming

1. A
2. C
3. D
4. A
5. D
6. C
7. A
8. B
9. D
10. A
11. D
12. C
13. D
14. B
15. C
16. B
17. A
18. C
19. B
20. A

Section 18
Assisting with urinary elimination

1. B
2. D
3. C
4. A
5. B
6. A

7. D
8. D
9. A
10. C
11. A
12. C
13. B
14. B
15. A
16. D
17. C
18. D
19. B
20. D
21. A
22. A
23. B
24. D
25. C
26. A
27. B
28. D
29. B
30. D

Section 19

Assisting with bowel elimination

1. D
2. A
3. D
4. D
5. B
6. A
7. B
8. A
9. C
10. D
11. A
12. D
13. C
14. B
15. A

16. C
17. A
18. A
19. C
20. D
21. B
22. B
23. C
24. D
25. A

Section 20

Assisting with nutrition and fluids

1. D
2. D
3. C
4. C
5. A
6. B
7. C
8. A
9. D
10. A
11. A
12. B
13. C
14. D
15. D
16. C
17. A
18. C
19. B
20. B
21. D
22. A
23. C
24. B
25. D
26. A
27. D
28. D

29. B
30. A
31. D
32. B
33. D
34. B
35. C
36. A
37. A
38. C
39. D
40. C

Section 21

Assisting with assessment

1. A
2. D
3. D
4. C
5. B
6. A
7. B
8. B
9. C
10. A
11. C
12. D
13. A
14. C
15. C
16. A
17. B
18. B
19. B
20. C
21. D
22. A
23. D
24. A

25. C
26. B
27. C
28. C
29. A
30. B
31. C
32. A
33. D
34. B
35. D
36. C
37. A
38. A
39. B
40. C
41. D
42. D
43. C
44. C
45. D

Section 22

Assisting with specimens

1. A
2. D
3. C
4. B
5. B
6. D
7. D
8. B
9. C
10. C
11. A
12. C
13. D
14. A
15. C

Section 23

Assisting with exercise and activity

1. D
2. A
3. A
4. B
5. C
6. D
7. A
8. B
9. C
10. B
11. C
12. A
13. A
14. C
15. D
16. A
17. D
18. B
19. C
20. B
21. A
22. C
23. A
24. D
25. C

Section 24

Assisting with wound care

1. D
2. B
3. C
4. A
5. D
6. B
7. C
8. C
9. A

10. D
11. A
12. C
13. A
14. B
15. C
16. A
17. B
18. C
19. A
20. D
21. C
22. A
23. D
24. B
25. C
26. A
27. D
28. C
29. B
30. D

Section 25

Assisting with pressure ulcers

1. A
2. A
3. D
4. C
5. B
6. D
7. C
8. B
9. D
10. A
11. B
12. C
13. A
14. B
15. D
16. C
17. A

18. C
19. D
20. D

Section 26

Assisting with oxygen needs

1. A
2. D
3. B
4. C
5. C
6. B
7. C
8. A
9. B
10. D
11. B
12. A
13. D
14. B
15. C
16. A
17. B
18. D
19. D
20. B
21. A
22. B
23. B
24. C
25. A

Section 27

Assisting with rehabilitation and restorative nursing care

1. C
2. A
3. D
4. B
5. C

6. A
7. D
8. B
9. A
10. C
11. D
12. C
13. D
14. A
15. B

Section 28

Caring for persons with common health problems

1. B
2. B
3. C
4. B
5. D
6. B
7. D
8. A
9. D
10. B
11. B
12. D
13. A
14. B
15. D
16. A
17. C
18. C
19. B
20. B
21. A
22. C
23. D
24. A
25. D
26. D
27. C
28. A
29. B

30. D
31. D
32. C
33. B
34. A
35. D
36. C
37. A
38. C
39. D
40. B
41. A
42. A
43. B
44. D
45. B
46. C
47. C
48. A
49. B
50. C
51. A
52. D
53. C
54. D
55. B
56. A
57. A
58. C
59. D
60. D
61. C
62. B
63. A
64. A
65. D
66. C
67. C
68. B
69. A
70. B
71. B
72. C
73. C

74. D
75. D
76. B
77. A
78. A
79. A
80. C
81. B
82. D
83. C
84. C
85. A
86. B
87. A
88. D
89. A
90. A
91. C
92. D
93. D
94. B
95. C
96. B
97. A
98. B
99. D
100.   C
101.   D
102.   D
103.   C
104.   A
105.   A
106.   D
107.   A
108.   D
109.   C
110.   B
111.   D
112.   A
113.   B
114.   C
115.   D
116.   D
117.   B

118.	B
119.	A
120.	C
121.	D
122.	A
123.	B
124.	D
125.	D
126.	D
127.	C
128.	B
129.	A
130.	B
131.	C
132.	A
133.	D
134.	D
135.	A
136.	C
137.	B
138.	B
139.	D
140.	D

Section 29

Caring for persons with mental health disorders

1. B
2. A
3. B
4. C
5. D
6. A
7. B
8. A
9. C
10. D
11. D
12. B
13. C
14. B
15. A

16. D
17. B
18. B
19. C
20. A
21. B
22. B
23. A
24. D
25. A
26. B
27. A
28. D
29. C
30. D

Section 30

Caring for persons with confusion and dementia

1. B
2. D
3. B
4. C
5. D
6. A
7. C
8. D
9. C
10. D
11. A
12. A
13. A
14. C
15. B
16. D
17. C
18. C
19. D
20. B

Section 31

Assisting with emergency care

1. A
2. A
3. D
4. C
5. D
6. B
7. D
8. A
9. C
10. B
11. D
12. A
13. B
14. D
15. C
16. B
17. D
18. C
19. C
20. A
21. D
22. B
23. A
24. C
25. D
26. D
27. C
28. A
29. B
30. B
31. B
32. A
33. C
34. D
35. C

Section 32

Assisting with end of life care

1. A

2. B
3. B
4. D
5. D
6. A
7. B
8. B
9. D
10. B
11. D
12. C
13. C
14. A
15. D

KEY POINTS EXAM PREP TEAM HAS NUMEROUS EXAM PREP MATERIALS.

SEARCH 'KEY POINTS EXAM PREP TEAM' ON AMAZON

FOR AUDIO BOOKS, SEARCH AUDIBLE.COM

.

www.ingramcontent.com/pod-product-compliance
Lightning Source LLC
Chambersburg PA
CBHW081149180526
45170CB00006B/1989